CHAIR YOGA
FOR SENIORS

CHAIR YOGA FOR SENIORS

STRETCHES AND POSES THAT YOU CAN DO SITTING DOWN AT HOME

LYNN LEHMKUHL

Skyhorse Publishing

Skyhorse Publishing books may be purchased in bulk at special discounts for sales promotion, corporate gifts, fund-raising, or educational purposes. Special editions can also be created to specifications. For details, contact the Special Sales Department, Skyhorse Publishing, 307 West 36th Street, 11th Floor, New York, NY 10018 or info@skyhorsepublishing.com.

Skyhorse® and Skyhorse Publishing® are registered trademarks of Skyhorse Publishing, Inc.®, a Delaware corporation.

Visit our website at www.skyhorsepublishing.com.

10 9

Library of Congress Cataloging-in-Publication Data is available on file.

Cover design by Tom Lau
Cover photo credit: Getty Images

Print ISBN: 978-1-5107-5063-0
Ebook ISBN: 978-1-5107-5065-4

Printed in China

For David. My forever partner. 144

TABLE OF CONTENTS

Preface   ix
Introduction   xi

PREFACE

Why did I write this book? As popular as chair yoga has become it is still hard to access. There are classes available but they are often limited to facilities that require membership. There are videos on YouTube, but they are unwieldy if you are trying to follow directions while not being close enough to your computer to actually see. And then, of course, there are books. Many of my private clients have asked me, over the years, to recommend a chair yoga book that they could use when on their own. In an effort to be as helpful as possible, I bought all of the chair yoga books I could find and read all of them, seeking the ideal one for seniors specifically. Sadly, I never found one that provides all of the elements that I believe to be essential. Either they are too complicated, use too much yogic vocabulary, have poses too difficult to execute, or are focused on spirituality instead of exercise. I never believed that any of the books I reviewed really understood what was required to motivate seniors to try, explore, and ultimately embrace an ongoing chair yoga practice. This is what led me to write the book that I believe is needed but did not exist until now.

My premise was simple and straightforward. Create a book for seniors that:

- Introduces them to easy-to-follow yoga practices.
- Presents material in an engaging and personal manner.
- Encourages readers to commit to a chair yoga routine.

- Reinforces the benefits to be derived from chair yoga.
- Create routines for seniors living with various maladies.

My goal for this book is also for readers to have fun. I strongly encourage readers to play music that they love while doing the poses. Music makes everything easier to do! That includes exercise.

I also have a great passion for sharing the personal joy that I experience when practicing yoga. By sharing this adoration, I want to express yoga's power of inclusion. Everyone can do it. There is no age, ailment, or body size that can't benefit from it. Yoga in a chair has opened its beneficial practices up to truly everyone. The fear of falling, which is on nearly every senior's mind, evaporates.

While I wrote this book, I felt inspired to include insights regarding the pursuit of a fulfilling a healthy lifestyle that go hand in hand with a yoga practice. I hope that when you read Chapter Eleven: I Feel So Much Better, I Want More! you will give thought to pursuing some, or all of my recommendations. I'll give you a sneak-peak. Chapter Eleven includes:

- The advantages of healthy eating.
- The benefits of meditation.
- The rewards of volunteering.
- The power of community and social connection.

My single most important message to you is to move. Set aside time each day to give your body and your mind the attention and care they deserve.

INTRODUCTION

I teach chair yoga to seniors who want or need to exercise while sitting down. The reasons for this are many. From being wheelchair-bound, to physical weakness, a neurological condition such as Multiple Sclerosis or Parkinson's disease, arthritis, balance issues, dementia, and the list goes on as to why many older people can only exercise while seated. Chair yoga is a great way for these people to stay active,

I have been practicing yoga for twenty years, and its benefits have been powerful. It has kept me flexible and strong in both body and mind.

During my many years as an advertising executive in New York City, I always managed to fit a yoga class into my hectic schedule. I traveled all over the country for work and would select hotel locations based on their proximity to yoga studios. The benefits I derived from my practice were an excellent motivator to stay focused and to stay healthy. Early in 2002, I decided to take a 200-hour yoga teacher training course to prepare for my life after corporate America. No small coincidence that the life-changing experience of being in New York City on September 11, 2001 helped guide me toward that decision.

I never looked back on my decision to prepare for my second career. I continued in the advertising industry for ten more years but always had my eye on my future life as a full-time yoga teacher. In 2013, I became increasingly aware of the fastest growing segment of the yoga market—chair yoga. As the Baby Boomer generation was aging, more and more seniors were looking toward sedentary exercise.

The combination of the rapid growth of the senior population along with the ever-increasing desire for health and wellness had led me to my calling: chair yoga for seniors! I sought additional training and found it with the pre-eminent chair yoga teacher Lakshmi Voelker. Lakshmi tours the country teaching the technique to registered yoga teachers. I was lucky to be able to study with her during her New York City training stint. In 2016, I completed my Adaptive Teacher Training, which is the therapeutic application of yoga. I now work full time serving the senior citizens of New York City. I offer seated low-impact yoga workouts in-home or on-site group sessions at senior homes, assisted living centers, and other organizations.

This book contains simple, easy-to-master techniques and exercises that I often teach to my clients. My hope with this book is to spread that knowledge.

CHAPTER ONE

WHY SHOULD I EXERCISE?

I wrote this book for every senior who wants a better life. Whether you are just starting an exercise program or continuing a lifelong practice, a regular exercise regimen will help you have a better life.

Consensus across all reputable news and medical sources agree that as a senior, engaging in physical activity is the single most important thing you can do to maintain mobility and independence. It will keep your muscles and bones strong, help with weight control and heart health, and aid proper joint function. The more you move, the better your strength and balance will be, and the less likely you will be to fall or lose the ability to perform basic daily functions. This is in addition to other health benefits of regular exercise, such as reduced risks of cardiovascular disease, type 2 diabetes, and certain cancers. Exercise even has positive effects on mood and may help improve cognitive function.

Let's get all of the facts out of the way. According to the Center for Disease Control and Prevention, the benefits of physical activity for seniors are many. They include:

- Helps maintain the ability to live independently.
- Reduces the risk of falling and fracturing bones.

- Reduces the risk of dying from coronary heart disease and of developing high blood pressure, colon cancer, and diabetes.
- Can help lower blood pressure in some people with hypertension.
- Helps people with chronic, disabling conditions improve their stamina and muscle strength.
- Reduces symptoms of anxiety and depression and fosters improvements in mood and feelings of well-being.
- Helps maintain healthy bones, muscles, and joints.
- Helps control joint swelling and pain associated with arthritis.

Every one of these points by itself is a great reason to start an exercise habit. But the first one on this list is a very critical one. It reduces the risk of falling!

Let's talk about falling. According to the Center for Disease Control and Prevention, falling is the leading cause of injury and death among adults aged sixty-five and older.

The *New York Times* reported on a recent study published in the *Journal of the American Medical Association* (*JAMA*) that revealed the rate of death for people seventy-five and older from falls more than doubled from 2000 to 2016. One of the speculated reasons for this is that people are living longer with illnesses that in the past they would have died from. Another reason likely to contribute to this rise is the increasing numbers of medications seniors take. Many of these drugs contribute to loss of balance and light-headedness.

Although the *JAMA* study is truly disturbing, falls are not inevitable. Fall prevention is a hot topic in newspapers, on the Internet, and on TV news programs. The recommendations are unanimous. They include safety installations in the home, removal of throw rugs, proper footwear, regular vision exams, good lighting, and the like. All of the lists recommend an exercise program. Dr. Lewis Lipsitz, a professor of medicine at Harvard Medical School and director of the Marcus Institute for Aging Research at Hebrew Senior Life, a housing, research, and health-care organization in Massachusetts, emphasizes the importance of incorporating exercise into a daily routine. He suggests exercising for at least twenty minutes a day. He recommends including weights in any routine, as they are very helpful in building strength in the legs.

Another expert in the field of elder care, physical therapist Michael Silverman, director of rehabilitation and wellness at Northern Westchester Hospital, talks about the impact of muscle decline in adults sixty-five and over. In an address, he noted that, "It affects the strength of the legs, hips, and core, all of which are critical to mobility and maintaining independence. The loss of muscle mass and strength in the arms can make it difficult to catch yourself if you do trip."

A 2016 comprehensive meta-analysis from the *British Journal of Sports Medicine* found that exercise alone reduces the risk of falls in older adults by an average of twenty-one percent and exercising three or more hours a week resulted in a thirty-nine percent decline in falls.

Though the risk of a fall increases significantly once people reach their eighties, researchers have found that people eighty-five and older in excellent health have no greater risk than someone twenty years younger.

Can we all agree that there is much well-documented information about the benefits of exercise for seniors? Yes! There is also a constant flow of information about the risks of falling. These two trending topics are resulting in widespread awareness amongst seniors, their caregivers, and their loved ones.

There is, however, one troubling result of the proliferation of falling statistics. The fear of falling has become an enormous concern among seniors. While a healthy dose of fear is fine—it can keep us alert to the dangers—it often crosses the line to become debilitating. Fear can also undermine you. Persistent worrying about a fall, if it's unwarranted, may cause you to limit your range of motion unnecessarily and cause you to avoid activities that you're capable of. It's estimated that a third to a half of older adults are concerned enough about potential falls that they have begun to restrict or avoid activities that would be beneficial for their health.

I am so happy to be a part of the chair yoga movement that helps seniors create for themselves a safe way to pursue health.

CHAPTER TWO

WHY CHAIR YOGA?

Yoga has been proven in numerous studies to improve one's balance, strength, and stability. As we age, our balance, strength, and stability deteriorate. These three losses are the main culprits behind the increase of falls that seniors experience. By practicing yoga, one can not only slow down the loss, but can also reverse the trend.

Yoga is truly for anyone of any age and ability. If you are strong and healthy, practicing yoga will help you stay that way. If you have health issues that are temporary or chronic, a gentle yoga practice will help you regain some of the strength and flexibility that has been compromised by your condition.

However, traditional yoga can be daunting to anyone who is not as steady on their feet as they once were, or to those who want to start slowly, or to anyone who would just feel more confident sitting down. Enter the chair! You can experience all of the benefits of yoga while seated. Chair yoga not only has all of the benefits of regular yoga, such as relieving stress, pain, and fatigue, but it can also help with joint lubrication, balance, and arthritis.

A key goal of yoga is restoring and maintaining the health of the spine. Poor posture interferes with the functioning of every part of our body. A rounded back restricts breathing and blood flow. With a regular yoga practice you can improve your posture by lengthening and strengthening your spine.

Another major benefit of yoga is the emphasis it places on feet. Feet are the foundation of your mobility. After years of wear and tear, most seniors experience occasional or sometimes chronic foot pain or numbness. This can lead to limited mobility, which is often a culprit in falling. A traditional yoga practice is done barefoot and works the foot throughout the routine. I have placed a major emphasis on the stretching and strengthening of feet in all of the routines.

In my practice, I have created easy to follow chair yoga routines for every level of fitness and experience. I share many of them in this book. My hope is that you will commit to making whichever routine you start with a habit. I believe that a regular practice of anything must be both enjoyable and easy to follow for it to stick!

Before I delve into the workouts, I want to tell you about some of my clients and friends to whom I have taught chair yoga and the impact it has had on their well-being. My interaction with these people has typically been private one-on-one sessions. Everything that I do or have done with them is part of one of the four programs that I lay out in this book. In my practice, I usually start with the Beginner Program but have advanced to the Intermediate in every one of the examples. There is of course a big benefit to having a yoga teacher personally guide you through the exercises. I have taken great care to present the material in easy-to-follow directions, so please have confidence in expecting similar results to those in the case studies below. Names have been changed to protect everyone's privacy.

MINDY: Wheelchair Bound and Suffers From COPD

Mindy is a retired psychotherapist in her eighties and suffers from numerous heart and lung ailments. Since spending the last five years confined to a wheelchair, she has gained a significant amount of weight. This of course exacerbates the symptoms of her conditions. Mindy's family reached out to me to come to her home and teach her chair yoga.

Mindy was receptive from the beginning. She desperately wanted to be restored to some semblance of her former self. We began each session by moving from her wheelchair to a dining room chair with arms. This was a laborious process. She had a substantial fear of falling during the transition. After many attempts to get up from the wheelchair Mindy would finally be on her feet and would very quickly hurl her body into the regular chair. She would achieve this move hunched over without standing up.

So from the beginning, I knew what we needed to work on first. Mindful breathing! Fear is a powerful force. When frightened, our breath becomes shallow, our shoulders tense up, and we experience a form of paralysis. Before we even started with the poses we focused on breath work to calm the nervous system. After a few weeks, the chair transition went slowly and smoothly. Within a few months Mindy was able to get up from the chair unaided and stand up straight for minutes at a time. She was able to sit with her head lifted, and her shoulders back and relaxed. This was a major achievement.

Mindy and I still work together. We spend a lot of time using dumbbells for upper body strength and doing leg and foot work to keep her muscles strong and flexible. Our long-term goal is for her to dance at her grandson's bar mitzvah!

PAULA: Suffers from Parkinson's

Paula has always been a very active woman. Now in her sixties, she spent decades as a high-powered executive and avid tennis player. Since being diagnosed five years ago with Parkinson's, she has had to make significant changes in her lifestyle. Paula is no stranger to yoga. She has enjoyed practicing for many years. Because she understands the health benefits of yoga, she was dismayed at how difficult it was becoming to get up and down from the mat. Paula's physical therapist recommended that she explore chair yoga. I worked with Paula for a few weeks to help her devise a program that she could do by herself in her home. She is now routinely doing the thirty-minute intermediate program that is described in this book and is thrilled with the results. She is experiencing increased mobility and strength in her arms and legs.

KAREN: Advanced Arthritis in Knees, Feet, and Spine

Karen is in her early seventies and still is a very busy lady! Two days a week, she babysits for her very active three-year old grandson, in addition to having a very active social life that includes activities like book club, knitting circle, and travel group. For the last decade, Karen has been plagued with arthritis in her knees, feet, and spine and it has definitely slowed her down. She had a knee replacement a few years ago and that helped her enjoy increased mobility. Karen never pursued a formal exercise habit, before or after the onset of her arthritis. She always rejected the idea for the most typical of reasons; she had no time! After her last trip with her travel group, she realized that she needed to explore exercise options. She was exhausted and in pain at the end of each day and was forced to skip some of the outings. This was a first for her. She wanted it to be the last. I convinced Karen to start a chair yoga routine. I promised her that it would be easy to follow, she could do it at home, and most importantly feel the benefits after a few short weeks. Karen wanted to start slow and I agreed with that choice. I knew if I presented her with anything too long or too difficult to understand or execute, it would be short lived. She did the short beginner program three times a week for three weeks and upped her time commitment to the thirty-minute routine after that. After six weeks, Karen was ready to try the intermediate twenty-minute routine. I knew that she was ready for it, especially the poses with weights. Karen is very happy with how this yoga habit has made her feel. She is living with more energy and less pain!

VALERIE: Recent Heart Attack Sufferer

Valerie is a lovely former school teacher in her mid-eighties who suffered a debilitating heart attack. Her daughter, upon the recommendation of Valerie's cardiologist, contacted me to come to their home to teach Valerie chair yoga. The physician felt strongly that Valerie needed a way to relieve her heightened anxiety since the attack. She was becoming increasingly reclusive, only going outside for doctor appointments. Valerie had always led a sedentary lifestyle, but since her heart attack, she rarely had the desire or energy to get off her couch. When I arrived at her home, she was very polite but clearly nervous. I could tell that she would rather being doing anything other than what we were about to do. My primary goal was to relieve her of her concerns. I made a promise to her that I know I kept. And it is the same promise I make to you the reader: I promise you that you will not hate this!

Now I knew that saying this would make her laugh, or at least smile. And it did. I explained that I always use music during my yoga sessions and that I liked to curate the song list to my clients' interests. She told me that she always loved Frank Sinatra but hadn't heard his music in years. I knew at that moment that this was going to work out well. Each week I would play Frank Sinatra on my phone, and Val sang along to every song. The time went by quickly for both of us. (I, too, love Frank!) Val slowly, but surely, gained strength and flexibility. We moved from the beginner moves I describe in this book to the intermediate poses much more quickly than I expected. By the third month we had incorporated weights. Val gained enough confidence, strength, and mobility to walk outside comfortably using a walker only for moral support.

LORETTA: Living with Lung Cancer and Recent Lung Surgery

Loretta's daughter, Diane, contacted me to come teach chair yoga to her mom. Loretta has lung cancer and had had half of her lungs removed two months prior to my arrival. She was on a portable oxygen machine and was generally weak, but had a strong desire to get back to her life as much as possible.

We started out extremely gently and took many breaks. She was filled with anxiety, as you can imagine, so we focused a lot of time on breath work. Slow and steady inhales and exhales calmed her body and mind. Her shoulders visibly relaxed as we went through the poses. Each time her breath quickened we would stop and wait until her regular breath was restored. In addition to strengthening her muscles, she learned to control her breath to restore balance and calm. This was a big deal for someone in her condition. I really enjoyed working with her because she was so determined to heal.

ROB: Long-Time Power Walker

In his thirties and forties, Rob was an avid runner. He ran five days a week for at least four miles on each outing. He would often say that he ran so he could eat whatever he wanted. After all, Rob was, and still is, a foodie! When he reached his fifties, Rob started to experience chronic lower back pain. He lived on ibuprofen, so he could continue to run. His orthopedist finally convinced Rob to replace running with power walking. He wasn't happy about the switch but dutifully transitioned. His back pain definitely eased, but was always lurking in the background. Rob has always maintained a healthy weight as a result of his decades of cardiovascular exercise. However, by the time he reached sixty-five he was experiencing ever-present stiffness and pain in his joints and back. He was beginning to stoop, and it took him extra time to get up out of a chair. What he failed to include in all of his years of running and walking was any flexibility and strength training. His excuse was always a lack of time.

But now that Rob is retired, he has lots of time. I am so happy that he has recognized the need to build strength in his body and work toward a flexible spine. I created a chair yoga program for Rob to do at home. He lives in Seattle, so I couldn't make house calls to check up on him. I was very happy to hear that he actually followed my recommendation to create a daily habit of strength and flexibility training. He has done so well with it that he sought out a class to join. Remember I said that he has a lot of time?

DAVID: An Avid Cyclist with Limited Flexibility in Spine and Shoulders

David is in his early seventies, and is still getting out on his fancy road bike, riding forty to sixty miles on any given day. He seeks out cyclists on his route who are half his age and wordlessly challenges them to a road version of a duel. He usually wins.

In his thirties, David was a marathoner; in his forties, he became a triathlete; and in his fifties, sixties, and now seventies, he focuses on his cycling. For decades, David has incorporated weight training into his fitness habit. But, much to my chagrin, he has not embraced a consistent flexibility habit and it shows. He has chronic shoulder, upper back, and neck pain. Imagine being in that tucked position on a bike for hours at a time! He has indulged in sporadic physical therapy visits or an occasional massage, but nothing consistent where he has to do the work, rather than someone working on him. I don't have a happy end to this story . . . yet! David is my husband and I am still trying to figure out how to get him to sit down and practice chair yoga!

Can you find yourself in any of these examples? I'm sure that you can. The variety of conditions and situations that these men and women have are representative of many seniors. I am so grateful that I found my way to these and many other seniors to help them invite an exercise program into their life. All, —except for David right now—have been changed for the better.

Now, let's make that happen for you.

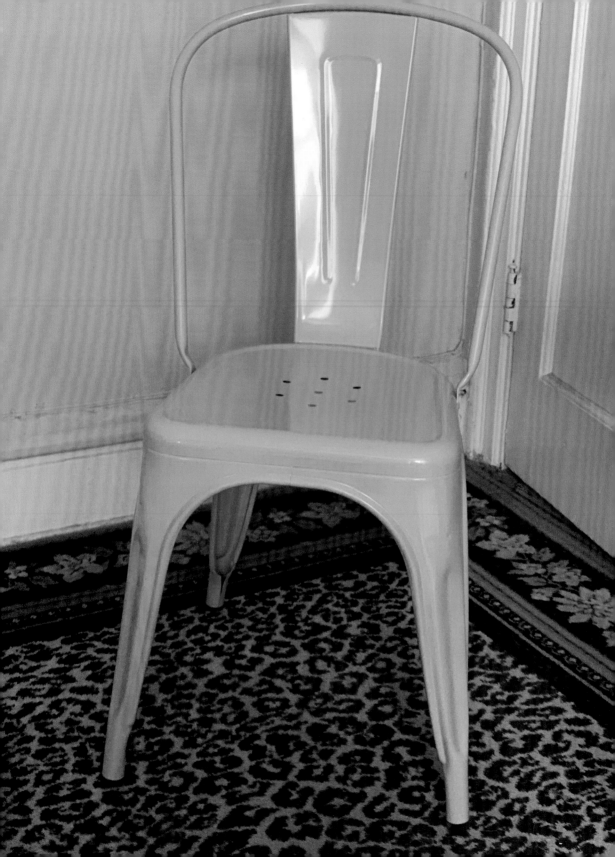

CHAPTER THREE

EASY TO DO AT HOME

WHAT DO I NEED?

The only essential equipment you will need if you are doing the beginner program is a straight-backed, non-cushioned chair. It can have arms or not. A folding chair or kitchen table chair is ideal. If you use a wheelchair, then you are good to go.

When you are ready to move on to the intermediate routines, you will require a set of two-pound dumbbells. These can be purchased at any sporting goods store or online.

WHERE SHOULD I SET UP?

I recommend that you create a space that you will want to come back to. You don't need a lot of room, but I do suggest that you find a space in your home that is uncluttered. Too many visual distractions will keep you from having a peaceful routine.

I highly recommend placing the chair in front of a mirror. This will provide you instant feedback on how you are executing the poses. Not essential, but very helpful.

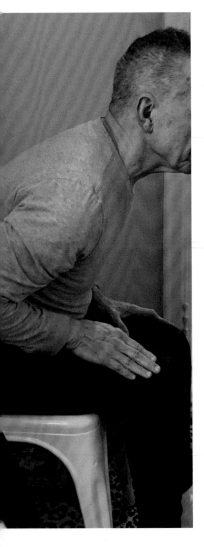

WHAT SHOULD I WEAR?

Dress in loose, comfortable clothes; wear nothing that will restrict your movement. If you are comfortable being barefoot, then do so. If you prefer the security of a shoe, then wear anything that has a rubber sole. Do not wear just socks on a hardwood floor. That will make it too slippery! If you are practicing on a rug, then socks are fine.

HOW SHOULD I PREPARE?

It is always a good idea to drink water before and after you exercise. Seniors notoriously drink too little water and are subject to bouts of dehydration. Don't eat for an hour before you start. You will be more comfortable if you don't have a full stomach.

WHAT TIME OF DAY IS BEST?

This depends entirely on you and your preference. When do you feel most energetic? I recommend the morning, but everyone has their own body clock. But what is more important than time of day is consistency. Pick an ideal time and stick to that. Research has shown that for something to become a habit, it is more likely to happen if you do it at the same time every day.

BEYOND THE ESSENTIALS

Music

I feel so confident that you are going to embrace this program and make it a part of your daily life that I am going to suggest ways to make this experience more pleasant. Let's begin with music! Music makes us feel good. It makes tasks seem less like work and more like fun.

But however you access music, whether via radio, CD player, or on your phone, please choose something that you enjoy. Choose something that makes you feel good. I have a chair yoga client who wants to listen to *La Traviata* exclusively and another who requests Pete Seeger. Give this some thought and select whatever is right for you.

Music Stand

A convenient tool when following an exercise routine from a book is to invest in a music stand. They are adjustable to eye level while seated, allowing you to have your hands free to move through the positions. Amazon has many to choose from for under $35.

WHICH PROGRAM SHOULD I SELECT? AND HOW OFTEN SHOULD I DO IT?

The answer may or may not be obvious. In case it isn't let's pick the right one for you.

If you never exercise or haven't in many years, I want you to start at the beginning with the beginner twenty-minute program. If you have exercised regularly in the past but are currently experiencing physical problems such as a chronic condition, recent surgery, or breathing issues, then by all means start at the beginning. The twenty-minute beginner routine is gentle, yet thorough. Each body part is worked. You most likely will not be sore the next day. If you can commit to doing it every other day, I promise that you will feel the positive effects after two weeks. By following my recommendations of creating an uncluttered, peaceful spot in your home to practice, wearing comfortable clothing, and listening to music that makes you feel good, I know that you will not think of four times a week as too much. After a period of three or four weeks, you can give thought to stepping up your commitment to the thirty-minute beginner program. If you are really feeling that the twenty-minute beginner routine has become too easy, then give some consideration to checking out the intermediate twenty-minute program.

What if you feel that you want to bypass the beginner program altogether and start with the intermediate twenty-minutes program? Then I heartily applaud your enthusiasm. If you are an active person without restrictive medical conditions, but just haven't made a commitment to a regular habit of exercise yet, then jump in! Nothing ventured, nothing gained, as they say. If it proves too demanding, you can always pull back, start at the beginning, and slowly but surely work toward it. The most important thing is that because you are reading this book, you have chosen to explore a way to a healthier, happier, and less anxious life. If someone gave this book to you as a gift and you are reading it so you don't appear ungrateful, then I assume the responsibility of earning your trust that this is the right way to go.

Do you suffer from osteoarthritis of the hands, knees, or hips? If so, you are in good company. One in three adults sixty-two and older have some form of it. If you haven't been exercising regularly then I suggest you check out the beginner arthritis program in Chapter Thirteen. It is gentle yet thorough in its attention to all of your joints. Once you have mastered the beginner program, move on to the intermediate one in Chapter Fourteen. It incorporates muscle strengthening around all of the affected joints.

Remember, whichever program you choose, it is only twenty to thirty minutes out of your day. Try to complete your program three to four times a week. You will not regret it.

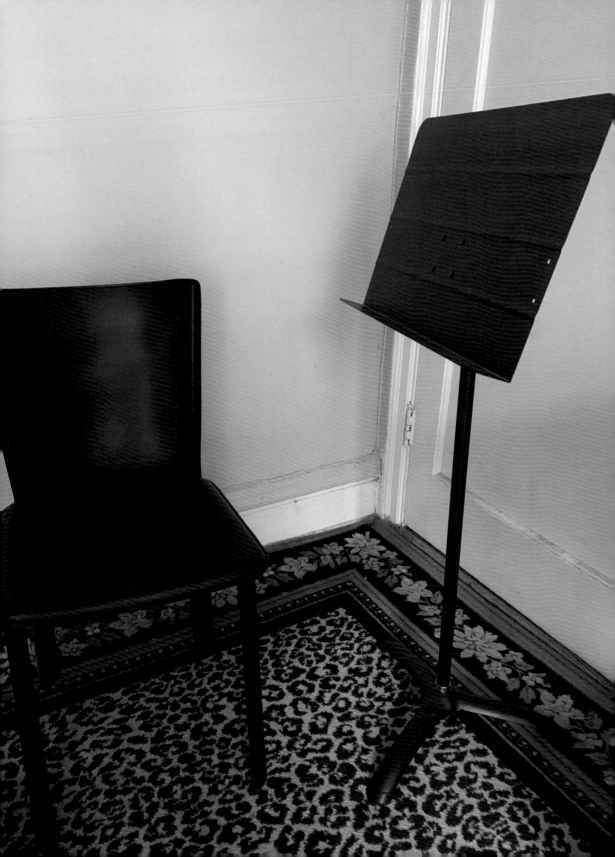

CHAPTER FOUR

WARMING UP

I always begin all sessions with five minutes of gentle warm-ups. Warm-ups prepare our bodies to stretch, and our muscles to lengthen, helping to avoid injury. An essential part of the warm-up is the breath. We humans, of course, are always breathing. We don't need to think about it at all in order to do it. What I am indicating here is mindful breathing where you take control of it to make it calm you and help you move with ease. I have often heard yoga teachers describe the mindful breath as the difference between exercise and yoga. I recognize that this is a difficult concept to understand at first, but I am confident that after you become comfortable doing the routines in this book you will understand and embrace the role of the breath. It is our power, our relaxer, and our protector.

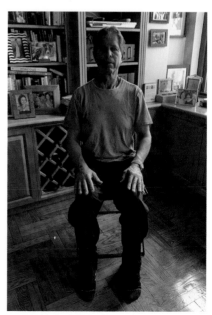

MOUNTAIN POSE

Starting Position: Sit up nice and tall in your chair, knees comfortably hip distance apart, with toes pointed straight ahead. Place your hands on your

Mountain Pose

thighs. Roll your shoulders up and then down your back and pull your navel to your spine. From this point on, when I refer to Mountain Pose, you will know that I mean to sit up tall in your chair, with your shoulders up, back, and down, knees hip distance apart, toes pointed straight ahead, and palms resting on your thighs. All chair yoga poses emanate from and return to Mountain Pose.

THE BREATH

Starting Position: Come to sit in Mountain Pose.

Movement: Take a slow and steady inhale through your nose, and a slow, steady exhale out your mouth. Don't force the breath. Try to make the exhale last as long as the inhale. You can start with a count of two on the inhale and a count of two on the exhale. If you can make each inhale and exhale longer, say a count of three to four, then go for it.

Repetitions: Take four complete breaths. Remember, slow and steady.

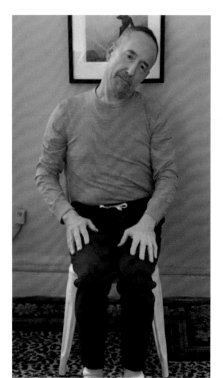

Side Neck Bend

Benefits: This type of breathing calms the nervous system and reduces anxiety. It prepares your body to move.

We will come back to these slow and healing breaths often throughout our sessions. Enjoy them! They make you feel good.

SIDE NECK BEND

Starting Position: Come to Mountain Pose.

Movement: Inhale to sit tall. As you exhale, drop your right ear to your right shoulder. Make sure that your shoulders are relaxed. Inhale to bring your head back to neutral. Now inhale to sit tall and exhale as you bring your left ear to your left shoulder. Inhale to bring your head back to neutral. That is one set.

Repetitions: Repeat the set three times.

Benefits: Stretches the sides of the neck.

20

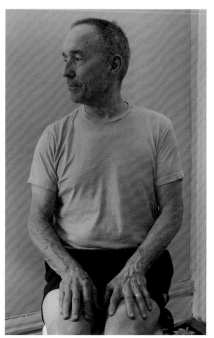

Neck Turns

NECK TURNS

Starting Position: Return to Mountain Pose.

Movement: On an inhale, very slowly turn your head to the right. As you exhale, very slowly return to center. On an inhale, turn your head slowly to the left. On a slow and steady exhale, return to center.

Repetitions: Repeat the set three times.

Benefits: Eases tension in the neck and helps to restore mobility in the upper back.

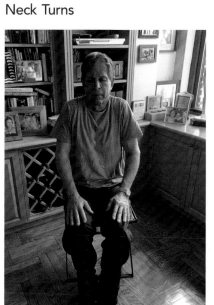

Shoulder Shrugs

SHOULDER SHRUGS

Starting Position: Resume Mountain Pose.

Movement: Inhale as you bring both shoulders up to your ears and exhale as you bring them back to neutral. Exaggerate the lift.

Repetitions: Repeat five times.

Benefits: Eases muscle tension in the neck and shoulders.

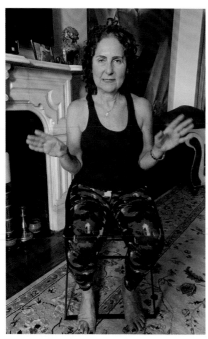

Wrist Circles

WRIST CIRCLES

Starting Position: Sit up tall in Mountain Pose. Sit with belly to spine and the crown of your head lifted toward the ceiling.

Movement: Keep your elbows close to the sides of your body and extend your hands in front of you. With fingers extended, roll your hands at the wrists. Wiggle your fingers as you roll your wrists.

Repetitions: Roll your wrists ten times, then switch direction and roll again ten times.

Benefits: Warms up the wrists and fingers. Also relieves inflammation in the hand joints.

ARM RAISES WITH BOTH ARMS

Starting Position: Assume Mountain Pose.

Movement: On a slow, steady inhale, raise both arms above your head. On a slow, steady exhale, lower your arms to starting position. Keep your shoulders relaxed during movement. If it is uncomfortable to raise your arms overhead, then raise them to a level that feels okay for you.

Repetitions: Repeat this five times.

Benefits: Encourages mobility in shoulder joints and strengthens arms.

Arm Raises with Both Arms

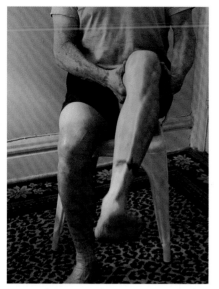

Knee Swings

KNEE SWINGS

Starting Position: Sit up tall in Mountain Pose, with belly in and shoulders back.

Movement: Clasp your hands under your right knee. Sit up tall with a straight spine. While holding under your knee, start to kick your leg out back and forth. This pose is one of the few that we do quickly. If you are unable to reach under your knee, then sit back in the chair and kick out your right leg, swinging back and forth with as much speed as is comfortable.

Repetitions: Do twenty times for each leg.

Benefits: Increases mobility and range of motion in the knees.

ANKLE CIRCLES WITH BOTH LEGS

Starting Position: Come to Mountain Pose.

Movement: On the inhale, lift your spine and extend both legs. Sit all the way back in your chair to achieve this pose. Keeping your legs as straight as you can, start to rotate your feet and ankles clockwise. The only body parts that move are your feet and ankles.

Repetitions: Rotate ten times in each direction.

Ankle Circles with Both Legs

Benefits: Promotes mobility in ankles and feet.

Your warm-up is complete. Your body is now ready for fifteen minutes of beginner yoga exercise, or twenty minutes if you choose the longer program. Regardless of the routine you select, do the same five-minute warm-up. In fact, if you only have a few minutes to exercise, do the five-minute warm-up. It is so much better than not doing anything at all.

CHAPTER FIVE

BEGINNER TWENTY-MINUTE FULL BODY PROGRAM

You have chosen to start your chair yoga exercise program with the twenty-minute program for beginners. Congratulations. I'm so happy that you are giving this a shot! As I once promised my client Valerie, you're not going to hate this!

I will repeat the warm-up instructions here so you don't have to go back and forth in the book. Remember the commitment I made to you the reader. Everything that follows is simple, easy to read, and easy to understand.

MOUNTAIN POSE

Starting Position: Sit up nice and tall in your chair, knees comfortably hip distance apart,

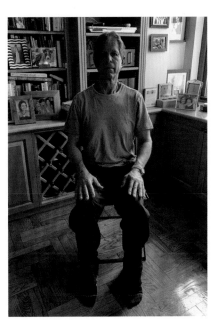

Mountain Pose

with toes pointed straight ahead. Place your hands on your thighs. Roll your shoulders up and then down your back and pull your navel to your spine.

THE BREATH

Starting Position: Come to sit in Mountain Pose.

Movement: Take a slow and steady inhale through your nose, and a slow, steady exhale out your mouth. Don't force the breath. Try to make the exhale last as long as the inhale. You can start with a count of two on the inhale and a count of two on the exhale. If you can make each inhale and exhale longer, say a count of three to four, then go for it.

Repetitions: Take four complete breaths. Remember, slow and steady.

Benefits: This type of breathing calms the nervous system and reduces anxiety. It prepares your body to move.

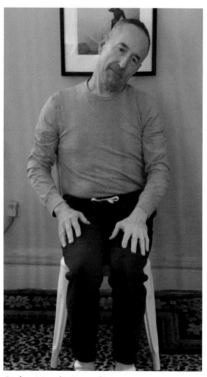

Side Neck Bend

SIDE NECK BEND

Starting Position: Come to Mountain Pose.

Movement: Inhale to sit tall. As you exhale, drop your right ear to your right shoulder. Make sure that your shoulders are relaxed. Inhale to bring your head back to neutral. Now inhale to sit tall and exhale as you bring your left ear to your left shoulder. Inhale to bring your head back to neutral. That is one set.

Repetitions: Repeat the set three times.

Benefits: Stretches the sides of the neck.

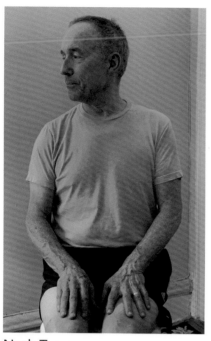

Neck Turns

NECK TURNS

Starting Position: Return to Mountain Pose.

Movement: On an inhale, very slowly turn your head to the right. As you exhale, very slowly return to center. On an inhale, turn your head slowly to the left. On a slow and steady exhale, return to center.

Repetitions: Repeat the set three times.

Benefits: Eases tension in the neck and helps to restore mobility in the upper back.

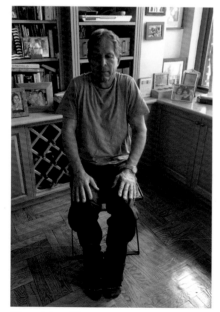

Shoulder Shrugs

SHOULDER SHRUGS

Starting Position: Resume Mountain Pose.

Movement: Inhale as you bring both shoulders up to your ears and exhale as you bring them back to neutral. Exaggerate the lift.

Repetitions: Repeat five times.

Benefits: Eases muscle tension in the neck and shoulders.

WRIST CIRCLES

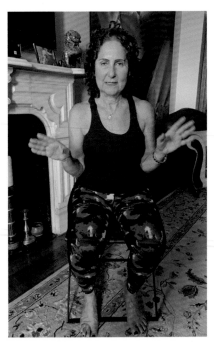

Starting Position: Sit up tall in Mountain Pose. Sit with belly to spine and the crown of your head lifted toward the ceiling.

Movement: Keep your elbows close to the sides of your body and extend your hands in front of you. With fingers extended, roll your hands at the wrists. Wiggle your fingers as you roll your wrists.

Repetitions: Roll your wrists ten times, then switch direction and roll again ten times.

Benefits: Warms up the wrists and fingers. Also relieves inflammation in the hand joints.

Wrist Circles

ARM RAISES WITH BOTH ARMS

Starting Position: Assume Mountain Pose.

Movement: On a slow, steady inhale, raise both arms above your head. On a slow, steady exhale, lower your arms to starting position. Keep your shoulders relaxed during movement. If it is uncomfortable to raise your arms overhead, then raise them to a level that feels okay for you.

Repetitions: Repeat this five times.

Benefits: Encourages mobility in shoulder joints and strengthens arms.

Arm Raises with Both Arms

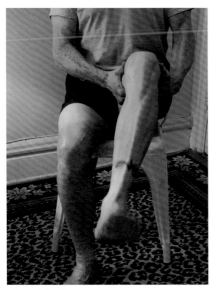

Knee Swings

KNEE SWINGS

Starting Position: Sit up tall in Mountain Pose, with belly in and shoulders back.

Movement: Clasp your hands under your right knee. Sit up tall with a straight spine. While holding under your knee, start to kick your leg out back and forth. This pose is one of the few that we do quickly. If you are unable to reach under your knee, then sit back in the chair and kick out your right leg, swinging back and forth with as much speed as is comfortable.

Repetitions: Do twenty times for each leg.

Benefits: Increases mobility and range of motion in the knees.

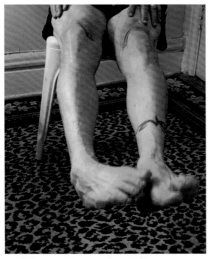

Ankle Circles with Both Legs

ANKLE CIRCLES WITH BOTH LEGS

Starting Position: Come to Mountain Pose.

Movement: On the inhale, lift your spine and extend both legs. Sit all the way back in your chair to achieve this pose. Keeping your legs as straight as you can, start to rotate your feet and ankles clockwise. The only body parts that move are your feet and ankles.

Repetitions: Rotate ten times in each direction.

Benefits: Promotes mobility in ankles and feet.

Your warm-up is complete. Let's pause and take three full breaths. Inhale slow and steady through your nose, and exhale slow and steady out your mouth.

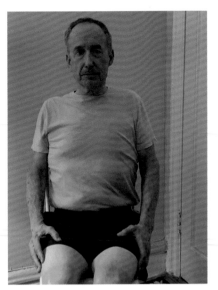

Shoulder Rolls

SHOULDER ROLLS

Starting Position: Sit up tall in Mountain Pose.

Movement: Inhale as you lift your shoulders up, then back, and exhale as you bring them around to starting position. Make the movement as smooth as possible, creating a continuous circle. After five slow and steady circles, reverse the movement. Lift your shoulders up on an inhale, bring them to the front of your body, and exhale as you bring your shoulders back to starting position. This direction always feels awkward. Don't worry, you are doing it correctly!

Repetitions: Repeat the movement five times in each direction.

Benefits: Opens up the shoulder joints and improves mobility.

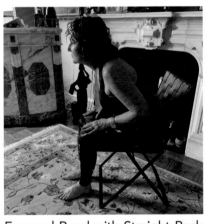

Forward Bend with Straight Back

FORWARD BEND WITH STRAIGHT BACK

Starting Position: Sit up tall in your chair with palms resting on your thighs.

Movement: On an inhale, bend forward from the hips, leading with your chin. Keep your spine straight. Go only as far as you can with your back straight. The bend is from the hips. On the exhale, come back up using your hands on your legs to push you back up. Look straight ahead throughout the movement. Do not look down. Depending on your spine's flexibility, this movement may be small. That is absolutely okay. Remember, the movement is slow!

Repetitions: Repeat each set five times.

Benefits: Expands mobility in the back and strengthens the muscles of the lower back.

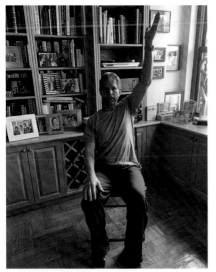
Alternating Arm Raises

ALTERNATING ARM RAISES

Starting Position: Come to Mountain Pose.

Movement: Inhale as you lift your right arm above your head, only if this movement is pain free. If it isn't, then lift your arm as high as it will go comfortably. Try to keep your extended arm straight and your shoulder relaxed. Exhale as you lower your arm down. Imagine that you are moving your arm through water. This image will help you move your arm slowly. Switch sides.

Repetitions: Repeat five times on each side.

Benefits: Lubricates the shoulder joint.

TORSO TWIST WITH ARMS UP

Starting Position: Sit up tall in Mountain Pose. Draw your belly in. Roll your shoulders up, back, and down your back.

Movement: Inhale as you lift both arms up as far as it is comfortable. Shoulders relaxed. Exhale. On an inhale, twist your upper body to the right. Arms stay up and hips and legs remain facing forward. Your head moves in the direction of the twist. On the exhale, come back to center. Keep your arms up. Now, inhale as you twist your torso to the left. Exhale back to center. After each set, return your hands to your lap.

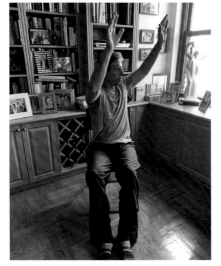
Torso Twist with Arms Up

Repetitions: Repeat each set of twists (a right twist and a left twist make up a set) five times.

Benefits: Tones the waistline (love handles) and promotes spine flexibility.

Let's pause here and take three full breaths. Inhale slow and steady through your nose, and exhale slow and steady out your mouth. Try closing your eyes during our breathing breaks. It helps to release tension.

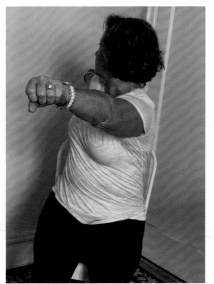

Torso Twist with Arms Extended Out to Sides

TORSO TWIST WITH ARMS EXTENDED OUT TO SIDES

Starting Position: Assume the Mountain Pose.

Movement: On an inhale, extend your arms out to the sides. Exhale. On an inhale, twist slowly to your right. Your head travels with your extended right arm. Exhale back to neutral. Don't lower your arms. If you are using a mirror, check to see that your extended arms are even and your shoulders are down. Inhale and twist to your left. Your head travels with your left arm. Return to neutral on an exhale and bring your arms down with hands resting on your legs.

Repetitions: Repeat each set of twists five times. Keep your arms extended throughout.

Benefits: Tones waistline and strengthens arms.

SIDE BODY LEAN WITH BOTH ARMS UP

Starting Position: Sit up nice and tall in Mountain Pose.

Movement: Inhale as you raise both arms up and stay. Exhale. On your next inhale, lean to your right. Exhale as you raise your arms back up to neutral. On a slow, steady inhale, with arms still up over your head, lean to your left. Exhale as you lift both arms up overhead. Make sure that your shoulders are relaxed and not hunched up toward your ears.

Repetitions: Do five sets. Arms stay up through-out exercise.

Benefits: Tones waistline.

Side Body Lean with Both Arms Up

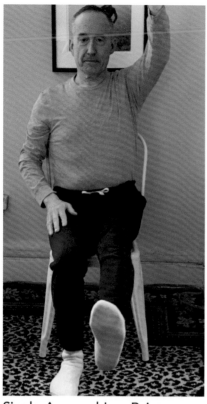

Single Arm and Leg Raises

SINGLE ARM AND LEG RAISES

Starting Position: Come to Mountain Pose.

Movement: Inhale as you lift your right arm and right leg together at the same pace, which is slow and steady. Exhale as you slowly lower your arm and leg.

Repetitions: Repeat five times on right side. Switch sides and repeat five times on your left side.

Benefits: Strengthens arm and leg muscles. Expands coordination.

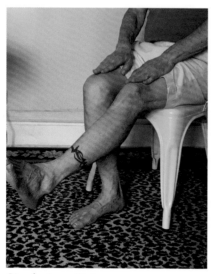

Single Leg Raises

SINGLE LEG RAISES

Starting Position: Come to sit tall in Mountain Pose.

Movement: Inhale as you lift your right leg from its bent position and exhale as you lower it back to Mountain Pose. Switch sides. This is a slow and controlled movement.

Repetitions: Repeat eight times on each side.

Benefits: Increases mobility in the knee joint.

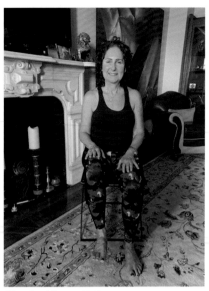

Single Knee Raises

SINGLE KNEE RAISES

Starting Position: Sit up tall in Mountain Pose.

Movement: Slowly lift your right knee straight up and slowly lower your foot to the floor. Lift your knee as high as you are able.

Repetitions: Repeat ten times on each side.

Benefits: Strengthens quadriceps.

Let's pause again and take three full breaths. Inhale slow and steady through your nose, and exhale slow and steady out your mouth.

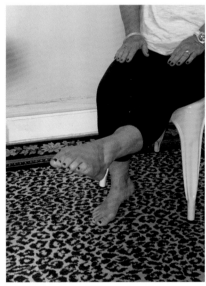

Single Leg Point and Flex

SINGLE LEG POINT AND FLEX

Starting Position: Sit tall in your chair with a straight spine.

Movement: On an inhale, extend your right leg straight out in front of you. Keeping your leg in this position, begin to point and flex your right foot. This can be done slowly or quickly. Either way, your foot and ankle get a terrific workout. Place your hands anywhere it is comfortable, whether that is down by your sides or in your lap. If possible, exaggerate both the point and the flex. When finished, return your foot to the floor and switch sides.

Repetitions: Repeat fifteen times on each side.

Benefits: Stretches shin and calf muscles while working the foot and ankle.

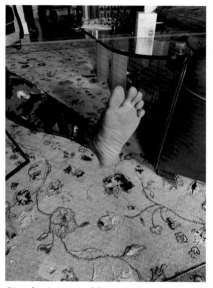

Single Leg Ankle Circles

SINGLE LEG ANKLE CIRCLES

Starting Position: Sit tall in your chair in Mountain Pose.

Movement: Inhale as you lift your right leg up and begin to rotate your foot clockwise. Slowly articulate the circles. Make them as big and exaggerated as possible. After about ten rotations, switch direction. Keep your lifted leg as straight as possible. Switch legs.

Repetitions: Do fifteen sets on each leg.

Benefits: Promotes mobility in and strengthens ankles.

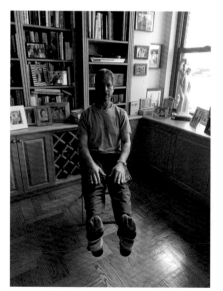

Both Legs Point and Flex

BOTH LEGS POINT AND FLEX

Starting Position: Sit in Mountain Pose.

Movement: On an inhale, extend both legs straight out in front of you. Keeping your legs in this position, begin to point and flex your feet. This can be done slowly or quickly. Either way, your feet and ankles get a terrific workout. Place your hands anywhere it is comfortable, whether that is down by your sides or in your lap. If possible, exaggerate both the point and the flex. When finished, return your feet to the floor.

Repetitions: Repeat fifteen times.

Benefits: Stretches shin and calf muscles while working the feet and ankles.

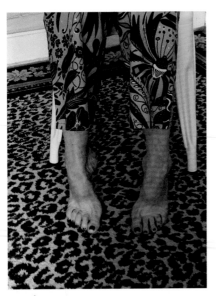

Heel Raises

HEEL RAISES

Starting Position: Sit tall and point feet straight ahead.

Movement: Keeping toes firmly planted on the floor, begin to lift your heels. Keep lifting your heels, making sure that your toes remain on the floor. If it is comfortable to do so, exaggerate the heel lift each time.

Repetitions: Repeat fifteen times.

Benefits: Stretches your calf muscles.

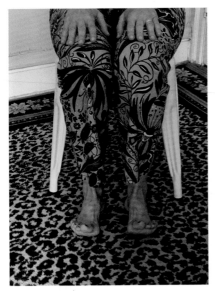

Toe Raises

TOE RAISES

Starting Position: Sit tall with feet pointed straight ahead.

Movement: Keeping heels firmly planted on the floor, begin to lift your toes. Keep lifting your toes while making certain that your heels remain firmly on the floor. Again, if it feels okay, exaggerate the lift each time.

Repetitions: Repeat fifteen times.

Benefits: Stretches the shins.

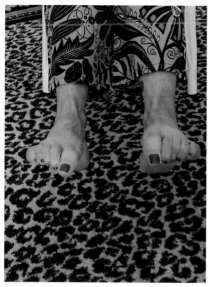

Toe Squeeze

TOE SQUEEZE/TOE SPREAD

Starting Position: Sit in Mountain Pose.

Movement: On an inhale, extend both legs out in front. Keep them there while you begin to scrunch your toes as tightly as you can, then release the squeeze and spread your toes out as widely as possible. Scrunch again, keeping everything tight, tight, tight! Then release and spread. Imagine that you can spread your toes so wide that no toe is touching another toe. This is really just a goal to work toward. Most likely, a toe or two will be touching.

Repetitions: Repeat this at least fifteen times. It feels good!

Benefits: Stretches toes, feet, and ankles.

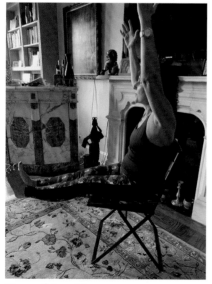

Everything Up

EVERYTHING UP!

Starting Position: This is your final Mountain Pose for this twenty-minute chair yoga workout. Make it a good one. Sit tall, knees hip distance apart, with toes pointing straight ahead. Keep your belly to spine.

Movement: On an inhale, slowly lift your arms and legs up at the same time. Try to keep all limbs and back as straight as comfort will allow. Exhale, and slowly return arms and legs to the starting position.

Repetitions: Repeat this pose five times.

Benefits: Strengthens full body.

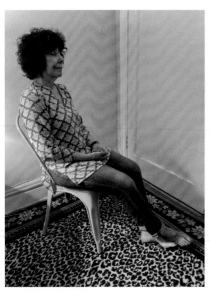

Deep Relaxation Pose

DEEP RELAXATION POSE

Starting Position: Lean back, resting your spine against the chair. Place your hands comfortably in your lap and close your eyes.

Movement: Breathe easily and relax your whole body. Allow any tension in your face, shoulders, legs, and feet to release.

Repetitions: Stay in this relaxed position for about five minutes, continuing to breathe naturally.

Benefits: Allows your body to absorb all of the benefits of your yoga practice.

Congratulations! You have finished your routine. I hope that you feel energized and relaxed. I urge you to plan on coming back to this very soon. Why not commit now to doing it every other day? The more of a habit it becomes, the faster you will experience the life-enhancing benefits of chair yoga.

And don't forget to drink some water. Your body needs it.

CHAPTER SIX

BEGINNER THIRTY-MINUTE FULL BODY PROGRAM

I'm so pleased that you have decided to commit to practicing chair yoga for thirty minutes. A few new poses will be introduced and we will increase repetitions for most of the poses that you did in the twenty-minute program. As always, we begin with a five-minute warm-up.

MOUNTAIN POSE

Starting Position: Sit up nice and tall in your chair, knees comfortably hip distance apart, with toes pointed straight ahead. Place your hands on your thighs. Roll your shoulders up and then down your back and pull your navel to your spine.

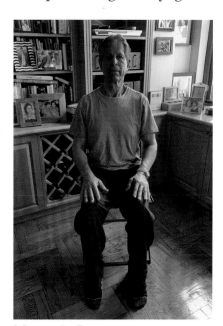

Mountain Pose

THE BREATH

Starting Position: Come to sit in Mountain Pose.

Movement: Take a slow and steady inhale through your nose, and a slow, steady exhale out your mouth. Don't force the breath. Try to make the exhale last as long as the inhale. You can start with a count of two on the inhale and a count of two on the exhale. If you can make each inhale and exhale longer, say a count of three to four, then go for it.

Repetitions: Take four complete breaths. Remember, slow and steady.

Benefits: This type of breathing calms the nervous system and reduces anxiety. It prepares your body to move.

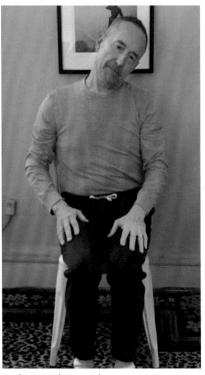

Side Neck Bend

SIDE NECK BEND

Starting Position: Come to Mountain Pose.

Movement: Inhale to sit tall. As you exhale, drop your right ear to your right shoulder. Make sure that your shoulders are relaxed. Inhale to bring your head back to neutral. Now inhale to sit tall and exhale as you bring your left ear to your left shoulder. Inhale to bring your head back to neutral. That is one set.

Repetitions: Repeat the set three times.

Benefits: Stretches the sides of the neck.

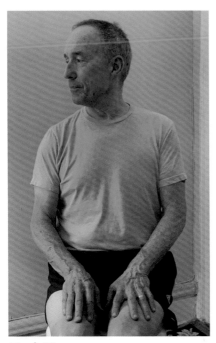

Neck Turns

NECK TURNS

Starting Position: Return to Mountain Pose.

Movement: On an inhale, very slowly turn your head to the right. As you exhale, very slowly return to center. On an inhale, turn your head slowly to the left. On a slow and steady exhale, return to center.

Repetitions: Repeat the set three times.

Benefits: Eases tension in the neck and helps to restore mobility in the upper back.

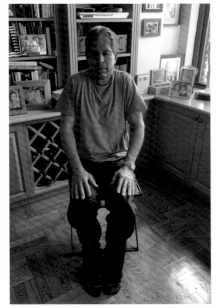

Shoulder Shrugs

SHOULDER SHRUGS

Starting Position: Resume Mountain Pose.

Movement: Inhale as you bring both shoulders up to your ears and exhale as you bring them back to neutral. Exaggerate the lift.

Repetitions: Repeat five times.

Benefits: Eases muscle tension in the neck and shoulders.

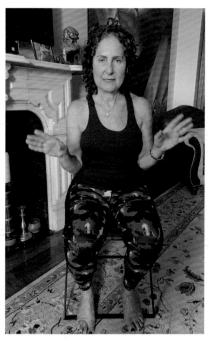

Wrist Circles

WRIST CIRCLES

Starting Position: Sit up tall in Mountain Pose. Sit with belly to spine and the crown of your head lifted toward the ceiling.

Movement: Keep your elbows close to the sides of your body and extend your hands in front of you. With fingers extended, roll your hands at the wrists. Wiggle your fingers as you roll your wrists.

Repetitions: Roll your wrists ten times, then switch direction and roll again ten times.

Benefits: Warms up the wrists and fingers. Also relieves inflammation in the hand joints.

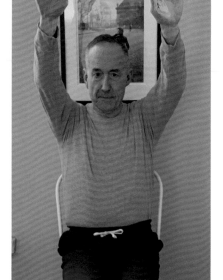

Arm Raises with Both Arms

ARM RAISES WITH BOTH ARMS

Starting Position: Assume Mountain Pose.

Movement: On a slow, steady inhale, raise both arms above your head. On a slow, steady exhale, lower your arms to starting position. Keep your shoulders relaxed during movement. If it is uncomfortable to raise your arms overhead, then raise them to a level that feels okay for you.

Repetitions: Repeat this five times.

Benefits: Encourages mobility in shoulder joints and strengthens arms.

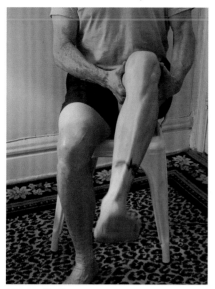

Knee Swings

KNEE SWINGS

Starting Position: Sit up tall in Mountain Pose, with belly in and shoulders back.

Movement: Clasp your hands under your right knee. Sit up tall with a straight spine. While holding under your knee, start to kick your leg out back and forth. This pose is one of the few that we do quickly. If you are unable to reach under your knee, then sit back in the chair and kick out your right leg, swinging back and forth with as much speed as is comfortable.

Repetitions: Do twenty times for each leg.

Benefits: Increases mobility and range of motion in the knees.

ANKLE CIRCLES WITH BOTH LEGS

Starting Position: Come to Mountain Pose.

Movement: On the inhale, lift your spine and extend both legs. Sit all the way back in your chair to achieve this pose. Keeping your legs as straight as you can, start to rotate your feet and ankles clockwise. The only body parts that move are your feet and ankles.

Repetitions: Rotate ten times in each direction.

Benefits: Promotes mobility in ankles and feet.

Ankle Circles with Both Legs

Our warm-up is complete. Let's begin!

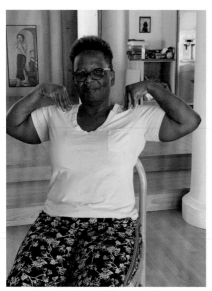

Hands on Shoulders Rolls

HANDS ON SHOULDERS ROLLS

Starting Position: Begin in Mountain Pose.

Movement: Place your hands on your shoulders and begin to make large circles with your shoulders, leading with your elbows. Breathe comfortably as you move. Switch the direction of your circles.

Repetitions: Repeat eight times in each direction.

Benefits: Warms up the upper back and releases tension in your neck.

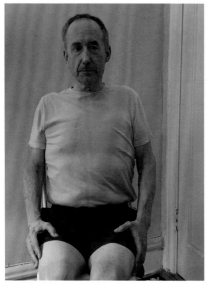

Shoulder Rolls

SHOULDER ROLLS

Starting Position: Sit up tall in Mountain Pose.

Movement: Inhale as you lift your shoulders up, then back, and exhale as you bring them around to starting position. Make the movement as smooth as possible, creating a continuous circle. After five slow and steady circles, reverse the movement. Lift your shoulders up on an inhale, bring them to the front of your body, and exhale as you bring your shoulders back to starting position. This direction always feels awkward. Don't worry, you are doing it correctly!

Repetitions: Repeat the movement five times in each direction.

Benefits: Opens up the shoulder joints and improves mobility.

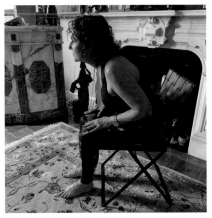
Forward Bend with Straight Back

FORWARD BEND WITH STRAIGHT BACK

Starting Position: Sit up tall in your chair with palms resting on your thighs.

Movement: On an inhale, bend forward from the hips, leading with your chin. Keep your spine straight. Go only as far as you can with your back straight. The bend is from the hips. On the exhale, come back up using your hands on your legs to push you back up. Look straight ahead throughout the movement. Do not look down. Depending on your spine's flexibility, this movement may be small. That is absolutely okay. Remember, the movement is slow!

Repetitions: Repeat each set five times.

Benefits: Expands mobility in the back and strengthens the muscles of the lower back.

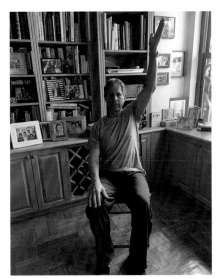
Alternating Arm Raises

ALTERNATING ARM RAISES

Starting Position: Come to Mountain Pose.

Movement: Inhale as you lift your right arm above your head, only if this movement is pain free. If it isn't, then lift your arm as high as it will go comfortably. Try to keep your extended arm straight and your shoulder relaxed. Exhale as you lower your arm down. Switch sides.

Repetitions: Repeat eight times on each side.

Benefits: Lubricates the shoulder joint.

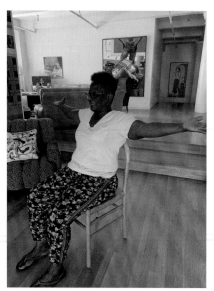

Extended Arms Palm Rotation

EXTENDED ARMS PALM ROTATION

Starting Position: Shoulders back and spine straight in Mountain Pose.

Movement: Extend both arms straight out to your sides with palms up. Keep arms in extended position with shoulders relaxed. Begin to move your palms to face down and then back to palms up. Nothing moves except your hands. Breathe normally throughout.

Repetitions: Do ten sets and return to Mountain Pose. Take an inhale and an exhale, then repeat movement for ten sets.

Benefits: Strengthens arms and warms up shoulders.

Extended Arms Hand Squeeze

EXTENDED ARMS HAND SQUEEZE AND SPREAD

Starting Position: Sit tall in Mountain Pose.

Movement: Extend both arms straight out to your sides. Take a slow, steady inhale as you squeeze your fingers into a tight fist, and exhale as you stretch your fingers out in an exaggerated way.

Repetitions: Repeat each set ten times. Return to Mountain Pose. Repeat movement for ten sets.

Benefits: Strengthens and stretches fingers and hands. It is an excellent workout for carpal tunnel sufferers.

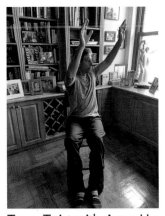

Torso Twist with Arms Up

TORSO TWIST WITH ARMS UP

Starting Position: Sit up tall in Mountain Pose. Draw your belly in. Roll your shoulders up, back, and down your back.

Movement: Inhale as you lift both arms up as far as it is comfortable. Shoulders relaxed. Exhale. On an inhale, twist your upper body to the right. Arms stay up and hips and legs remain facing forward. Your head moves in the direction of the twist. On the exhale, come back to center. Keep your arms up. Now, inhale as you twist your torso to the left. Exhale back to center. After each set, return your hands to your lap.

Repetitions: Repeat each set of twists (a right twist and a left twist make up a set) eight times.

Benefits: Tones the waistline (love handles) and promotes spine flexibility.

Let's pause here and take three full breaths. Inhale slow and steady through your nose, and exhale slow and steady out your mouth. Try closing your eyes during our breathing breaks. It helps to release tension.

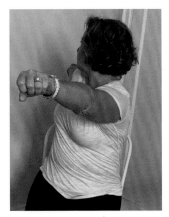

Torso Twist with Arms Extended Out to Sides

TORSO TWIST WITH ARMS EXTENDED OUT TO SIDES

Starting Position: Assume the Mountain Pose.

Movement: On an inhale, extend your arms out to the sides. Exhale. On an inhale, twist slowly to your right. Your head travels with your extended right arm. Exhale back to neutral. Don't lower your arms. If you are using a mirror, check to see that your extended arms are even and your shoulders are down. Inhale and twist to your left. Your head travels with your left arm. Return to neutral on an exhale and bring your arms down with hands resting on your legs.

Repetitions: Repeat each set eight times.

Benefits: Tones waistline and strengthens arms.

BACK BEND

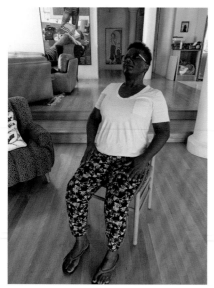

Back Bend

Starting Position: Come to Mountain Pose.

Movement: Rest your hands with your palms down on your legs. On a slow, steady inhale, lift your chest, arch your back slightly, open up your shoulders, and gaze up to the ceiling. On your exhale, slowly drop your head, round your back and shoulders, and gaze down at the floor. Now return to neutral. Let's do that again. Make the four movements—lift chest, arch back, open shoulders, and gaze up—happen simultaneously on a single inhale and likewise on the exhale. This may take a bit of practice but is worth the effort.

Repetitions: Do five sets of this pose.

Benefits: Warms up the thoracic and lumbar spine (upper and lower back). Promotes good posture.

SIDE BODY LEAN WITH BOTH ARMS UP

Starting Position: Sit up nice and tall in Mountain Pose.

Movement: Inhale as you raise both arms up and stay. Exhale. On your next inhale, lean to your right. Exhale as you raise your arms back up to neutral. On a slow, steady inhale, with arms still up over your head, lean to your left. Exhale as you lift both arms up overhead. Make sure that your shoulders are relaxed and not hunched up toward your ears.

Repetitions: Do eight sets. Arms stay up throughout exercise. On the last rep on each side, hold the pose and take one full breath. Release pose and return to neutral.

Benefits: Tones waistline.

Side Body Lean with Both Arms Up

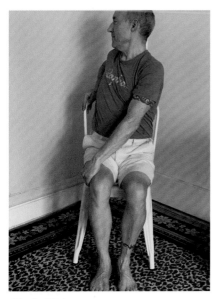

Chair Twist

CHAIR TWIST

Starting Position: Sit tall with feet hip distance apart.

Movement: Slowly twist your upper torso to your right and put your right hand on the top of the back of the chair. Place your left hand on the outside of your right knee. Make sure that both of your knees are pointing straight ahead. On an inhale, lift your spine and then exhale as you slowly twist to the right. Come back to neutral. This pose takes some practice. Do make sure that your lower body stays still!

Repetitions: Repeat five times on each side.

Benefits: Massages internal organs and tones the waistline.

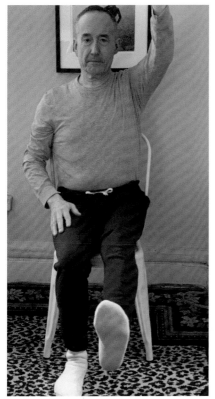

SINGLE ARM AND LEG RAISES

Starting Position: Come to Mountain Pose.

Movement: Inhale as you lift your right arm and right leg together at the same pace, which is slow and steady. Exhale as you slowly lower your arm and leg.

Repetitions: Repeat ten times on each side.

Benefits: Strengthens arm and leg muscles. Expands coordination.

Single Arm and Leg Raises

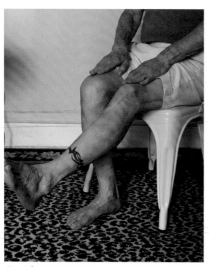

Single Leg Raises

SINGLE LEG RAISES

Starting Position: Come to sit tall in Mountain Pose.

Movement: Inhale as you lift your right leg from its bent position and exhale as you lower it back to Mountain Pose. Switch sides. This is a slow and controlled movement.

Repetitions: Repeat ten times on each side.

Benefits: Increases mobility in the knee joint.

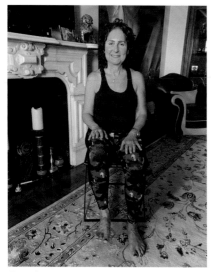

Single Knee Raises

SINGLE KNEE RAISES

Starting Position: Sit up tall in Mountain Pose.

Movement: Slowly lift your right knee straight up and slowly lower your foot to the floor. Lift your knee as high as you are able.

Repetitions: Repeat ten times on each side.

Benefits: Strengthens quadriceps.

Let's pause again and take three full breaths. Inhale slow and steady through your nose, and exhale slow and steady out your mouth.

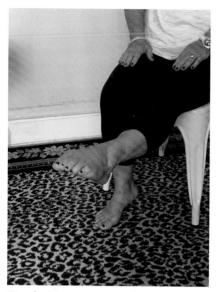

Single Leg Point and Flex

SINGLE LEG POINT AND FLEX

Starting Position: Sit tall in your chair with a straight spine.

Movement: On an inhale, extend your right leg straight out in front of you. Keeping your leg in this position, begin to point and flex your right foot. This can be done slowly or quickly. Either way, your foot and ankle get a terrific workout. Place your hands anywhere it is comfortable, whether that is down by your sides or in your lap. If possible, exaggerate both the point and the flex. When finished, return your foot to the floor and switch sides.

Repetitions: Repeat fifteen times on each side.

Benefits: Stretches shin and calf muscles while working the foot and ankle.

SINGLE LEG ANKLE CIRCLES

Starting Position: Sit tall in your chair in Mountain Pose.

Movement: Inhale as you lift your right leg up and begin to rotate your foot clockwise. Slowly articulate the circles. Make them as big and exaggerated as possible. After about ten rotations, switch direction. Keep your lifted leg as straight as possible. Switch legs.

Repetitions: Ten sets each side.

Benefits: Promotes mobility in and strengthens ankles.

Single Leg Ankle Circles

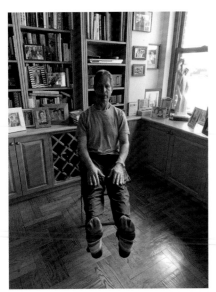
Both Legs Point and Flex

BOTH LEGS POINT AND FLEX

Starting Position: Sit in Mountain Pose.

Movement: On an inhale, extend both legs straight out in front of you. Keeping your legs in this position, begin to point and flex your feet. This can be done slowly or quickly. Either way, your feet and ankles get a terrific workout. Place your hands anywhere it is comfortable, whether that is down by your sides or in your lap. If possible, exaggerate both the point and the flex. When finished, return your feet to the floor.

Repetitions: Repeat fifteen times.

Benefits: Stretches shin and calf muscles while working the feet and ankles.

HEEL RAISES

Starting Position: Sit tall and point feet straight ahead.

Movement: Keeping toes firmly planted on the floor, begin to lift your heels. Keep lifting your heels, making sure that your toes remain on the floor. If it is comfortable to do so, exaggerate the heel lift each time.

Repetitions: Repeat fifteen times.

Benefits: Stretches your calf muscles.

Heel Raises

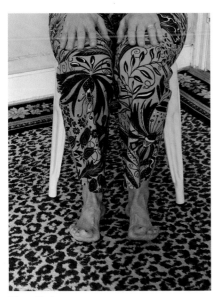

Toe Raises

TOE RAISES

Starting Position: Sit tall with feet pointed straight ahead.

Movement: Keeping heels firmly planted on the floor, begin to lift your toes. Keep lifting your toes while making certain that your heels remain firmly on the floor. Again, if it feels okay, exaggerate the lift each time.

Repetitions: Repeat fifteen times.

Benefits: Stretches the shins.

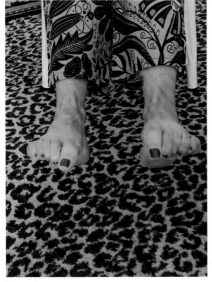

Toe Squeeze

TOE SQUEEZE/TOE SPREAD

Starting Position: Sit in Mountain Pose.

Movement: On an inhale, extend both legs out in front. Keep them there while you begin to scrunch your toes as tightly as you can, then release the squeeze and spread your toes out as widely as possible. Scrunch again, keeping everything tight, tight, tight! Then release and spread. Imagine that you can spread your toes so wide that no toe is touching another toe. This is really just a goal to work toward. Most likely, a toe or two will be touching.

Repetitions: Repeat this at least fifteen times. It feels good!

Benefits: Stretches toes, feet, and ankles.

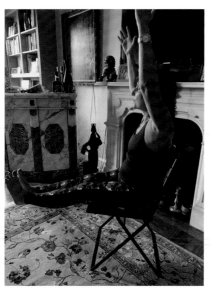

Everything Up

EVERYTHING UP!

Starting Position: This is your final Mountain Pose for this thirty-minute chair yoga workout. Make it a good one. Sit tall, knees hip distance apart, with toes pointing straight ahead. Keep your belly to spine.

Movement: On an inhale, slowly lift your arms and legs up at the same time. Try to keep all limbs and back as straight as comfort will allow. Exhale, and slowly return arms and legs to the starting position.

Repetitions: Repeat this pose eight times.

Benefits: Strengthens full body.

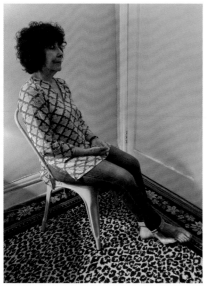

Deep Relaxation Pose

DEEP RELAXATION POSE

Starting Position: Lean back, resting your spine against the chair. Place your hands comfortably in your lap and close your eyes.

Movement: Breathe easily and relax your whole body. Allow any tension in your face, shoulders, legs, and feet to release.

Repetitions: Stay in this relaxed position for about five minutes, continuing to breathe naturally.

Benefits: Allows your body to absorb all of the benefits of your yoga practice.

You are finished for the day! Drink some water and enjoy the satisfaction that you are taking good care of yourself.

CHAPTER SEVEN

INTERMEDIATE TWENTY-MINUTE FULL BODY PROGRAM

Whether you are starting at the intermediate level or have graduated to it after spending some quality time at the beginner program, I welcome you to this new commitment level. In this routine, we are going to increase the difficulty of the moves, but in a safe and achievable way. The only new equipment you will need are two two-pound dumbbells. Many of my students who start out working with two-pound weights graduate to three- or even four-pound weights after a few months of practicing three to five times a week. Just tuck this info away for future consideration.

I want to remind you of a few items on our getting started checklist:

- Drink a glass of water.
- Dress comfortably.
- Have your favorite music ready to go.
- Place your chair in an uncluttered space.
- Be barefoot or wear rubber soled shoes on any floor surface. Wear socks only on carpet.

- Place this book on your music stand. It is really helpful to have the book at eye level.
- Place dumbbells within easy reach.

We are ready to begin! Let's do our warm-up.

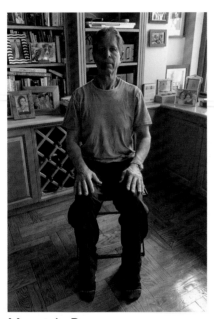

Mountain Pose

MOUNTAIN POSE

Starting Position: Sit up nice and tall in your chair, knees comfortably hip distance apart, with toes pointed straight ahead. Place your hands on your thighs. Roll your shoulders up and then down your back and pull your navel to your spine.

THE BREATH

Starting Position: Come to sit in Mountain Pose.

Movement: Take a slow and steady inhale through your nose, and a slow, steady exhale out your mouth. Don't force the breath. Try to make the exhale last as long as the inhale. You can start with a count of two on the inhale and a count of two on the exhale. If you can make each inhale and exhale longer, say a count of three to four, then go for it.

Repetitions: Take four complete breaths. Remember, slow and steady.

Benefits: This type of breathing calms the nervous system and reduces anxiety. It prepares your body to move.

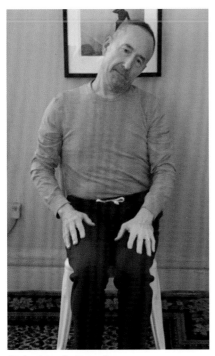

Side Neck Bend

SIDE NECK BEND

Starting Position: Come to Mountain Pose.

Movement: Inhale to sit tall. As you exhale, drop your right ear to your right shoulder. Make sure that your shoulders are relaxed. Inhale to bring your head back to neutral. Now inhale to sit tall and exhale as you bring your left ear to your left shoulder. Inhale to bring your head back to neutral. That is one set.

Repetitions: Repeat the set three times.

Benefits: Stretches the sides of the neck.

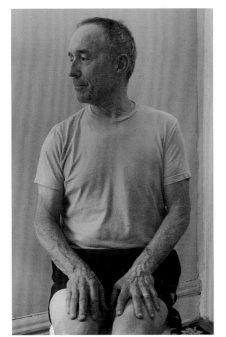

Neck Turns

NECK TURNS

Starting Position: Return to Mountain Pose.

Movement: On an inhale, very slowly turn your head to the right. As you exhale, very slowly return to center. On an inhale, turn your head slowly to the left. On a slow and steady exhale, return to center.

Repetitions: Repeat the set three times.

Benefits: Eases tension in the neck and helps to restore mobility in the upper back.

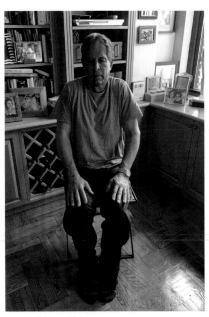

Shoulder Shrugs

SHOULDER SHRUGS

Starting Position: Resume Mountain Pose.

Movement: Inhale as you bring both shoulders up to your ears and exhale as you bring them back to neutral. Exaggerate the lift.

Repetitions: Repeat five times.

Benefits: Eases muscle tension in the neck and shoulders.

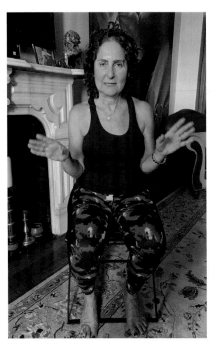

Wrist Circles

WRIST CIRCLES

Starting Position: Sit up tall in Mountain Pose. Sit with belly to spine and the crown of your head lifted toward the ceiling.

Movement: Keep your elbows close to the sides of your body and extend your hands in front of you. With fingers extended, roll your hands at the wrists. Wiggle your fingers as you roll your wrists.

Repetitions: Roll your wrists ten times, then switch direction and roll again ten times.

Benefits: Warms up the wrists and fingers. Also relieves inflammation in the hand joints.

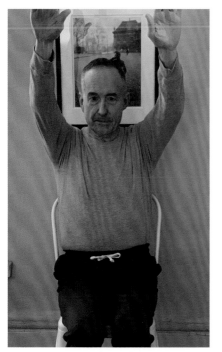

Arm Raises with Both Arms

ARM RAISES WITH BOTH ARMS

Starting Position: Assume Mountain Pose.

Movement: On a slow, steady inhale, raise both arms above your head. On a slow, steady exhale, lower your arms to starting position. Keep your shoulders relaxed during movement. If it is uncomfortable to raise your arms overhead, then raise them to a level that feels okay for you.

Repetitions: Repeat this five times.

Benefits: Encourages mobility in shoulder joints and strengthens arms.

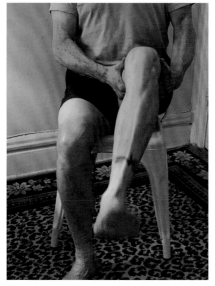

Knee Swings

KNEE SWINGS

Starting Position: Sit up tall in Mountain Pose, with belly in and shoulders back.

Movement: Clasp your hands under your right knee. Sit up tall with a straight spine. While holding under your knee, start to kick your leg out back and forth. This pose is one of the few that we do quickly. If you are unable to reach under your knee, then sit back in the chair and kick out your right leg, swinging back and forth with as much speed as is comfortable.

Repetitions: Do twenty times for each leg.

Benefits: Increases mobility and range of motion in the knees.

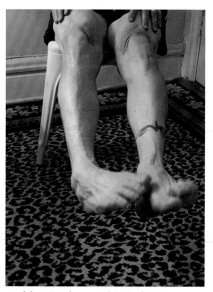

Ankle Circles with Both Legs

ANKLE CIRCLES WITH BOTH LEGS

Starting Position: Come to Mountain Pose.

Movement: On the inhale, lift your spine and extend both legs. Sit all the way back in your chair to achieve this pose. Keeping your legs as straight as you can, start to rotate your feet and ankles clockwise. The only body parts that move are your feet and ankles.

Repetitions: Rotate ten times in each direction.

Benefits: Promotes mobility in ankles and feet.

We are finished with our warm-up. Let's begin our chair yoga practice.

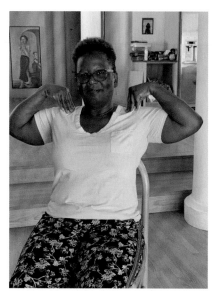

Hands on Shoulders Rolls

HANDS ON SHOULDERS ROLLS

Starting Position: Begin in Mountain Pose.

Movement: Place your hands on your shoulders and begin to make large circles with your shoulders, leading with your elbows. Breathe comfortably as you move. Switch the direction of your circles.

Repetitions: Repeat eight times in each direction.

Benefits: Warms up the upper back and releases tension in your neck.

60

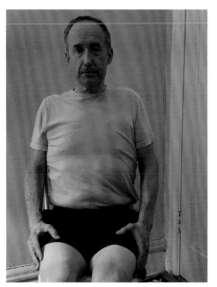

Shoulder Rolls

SHOULDER ROLLS

Starting Position: Sit up tall in Mountain Pose.

Movement: Inhale as you lift your shoulders up, then back, and exhale as you bring them around to starting position. Make the movement as smooth as possible, creating a continuous circle. After five slow and steady circles, reverse the movement. Lift your shoulders up on an inhale, bring them to the front of your body, and exhale as you bring your shoulders back to starting position. This direction always feels awkward. Don't worry, you are doing it correctly!

Repetitions: Repeat the movement eight times in each direction.

Benefits: Opens up the shoulder joints and improves mobility.

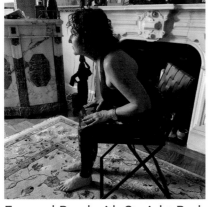

Forward Bend with Straight Back

FORWARD BEND WITH STRAIGHT BACK

Starting Position: Sit up tall in your chair with palms resting on your thighs.

Movement: On an inhale, bend forward from the hips, leading with your chin. Keep your spine straight. Go only as far as you can with your back straight. The bend is from the hips. On the exhale, come back up using your hands on your legs to push you back up. Look straight ahead throughout the movement. Do not look down. Depending on your spine's flexibility, this movement may be small. That is absolutely okay. Remember, the movement is slow!

Repetitions: Repeat eight times. On the eighth rep, hold bent position and take one full breath consisting of a slow, steady inhale and a slow, steady exhale. Return to neutral.

Benefits: Expands mobility in the back and strengthens the muscles of the lower back.

61

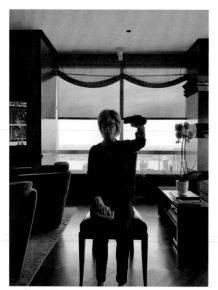

Alternating Arm Raises with Weights

ALTERNATING ARM RAISES WITH WEIGHTS

Starting Position: Come to Mountain Pose holding the two-pound weights in your hands as they rest on your thighs.

Movement: Inhale as you lift your right arm above your head, only if this movement is pain free. If it isn't, then lift your arm as high as it will go comfortably. Try to keep your extended arm straight and your shoulder relaxed. Exhale as you lower your arm down. Switch sides.

Repetitions: Repeat six times on each side. Hold the pose on the last rep of each side and take one full breath. Release pose and return to neutral. You are holding the weights in both hands throughout the exercise.

Benefits: Lubricates the shoulder joint and strengthens the arms.

TORSO TWIST WITH ARMS EXTENDED WITH WEIGHTS

Starting Position: Assume the Mountain Pose with weights in each hand.

Movement: Hold a weight in each hand and on an inhale, extend your arms out to the sides. Exhale. On an inhale, twist slowly to your right. Your head travels with your extended right arm. Exhale back to neutral. Don't lower your arms. If you are using a mirror, check to see that your extended arms are even and that your shoulders are down. Inhale and twist to

Torso Twist with Arms Extended with Weights

your left. Your head travels with your left arm. Return to neutral and bring your arms down with hands resting on your legs.

Repetitions: Repeat each set eight times. Hold the pose on the last rep on each side and take one full breath. Release pose and return to neutral.

Benefits: Tones waistline and strengthens arms.

Let's pause and take three full breaths. Inhale slow and steady through your nose, and exhale slow and steady out your mouth.

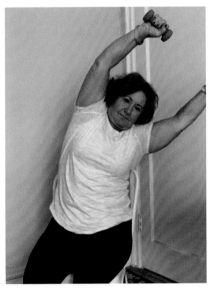

Side Body Lean with Weights

SIDE BODY LEAN WITH WEIGHTS

Starting Position: Sit up nice and tall in Mountain Pose. Take weights in each hand and rest them on your thighs.

Movement: With weights in both hands, inhale as you lift both arms up and stay. Exhale. On your next inhale, lean to your right. Exhale as you lift your arms back up to neutral. On a slow, steady inhale, with arms still up over your head, lean to your left. Exhale as you lift both arms back up overhead.

Repetitions: Do eight sets. Arms stay up throughout. On the last rep on each side, hold the pose and take one full breath. Release pose and return to neutral.

Benefits: Tones waistline.

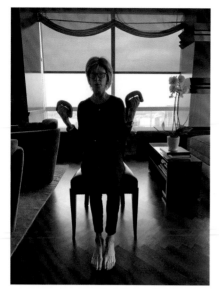

Bicep Curls Alternating Arms with Weights

BICEP CURLS ALTERNATING ARMS WITH WEIGHTS

Starting Position: Come to sit in Mountain Pose with the weights in your hands.

Movement: Drop your arms by your sides. Keep your elbows glued to the sides of your body. On the inhale, slowly bend your right arm up and exhale as you lower it down to starting position. Inhale as you bring the left arm up and exhale to bring it back to start. Your elbows never leave the sides of your torso during the movement.

Repetitions: Repeat eight times on each side. Pause for a breath and repeat the exercise for eight reps on each side.

Benefits: Builds muscle in the biceps.

SINGLE ARM AND LEG RAISES WITH WEIGHTS

Starting Position: Come to Mountain Pose with weights resting in your lap.

Movement: Inhale as you lift your right arm (weight is in your hand) and right leg together. Both arm and leg should be as straight as you can make them. Exhale as you lower them.

Repetitions: Repeat six times on each side. Hold pose in the up position on the last rep of each side and take one full breath (an inhale and an exhale). Release the pose and return to neutral.

Benefits: Strengthens arm and leg muscles. Expands coordination.

Single Arm and Leg Raises with Weights

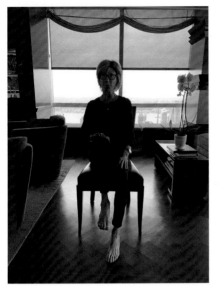

Single Knee Raises with Weights

SINGLE KNEE RAISES WITH WEIGHTS

Starting Position: Sit up tall in Mountain Pose with both weights resting on the top of your right knee.

Movement: Resting your right hand over the two weights to hold them in place, slowly lift your right knee straight up and then slowly lower your foot to the floor. Repeat ten times. On the final rep, hold your knee up and take one full breath. Return your foot to the floor and switch sides. Place the two weights on top of your left knee.

Repetitions: Repeat ten times on each side. Make sure that you take one full breath on the last rep of each side. Release pose.

Benefits: Strengthens quadriceps.

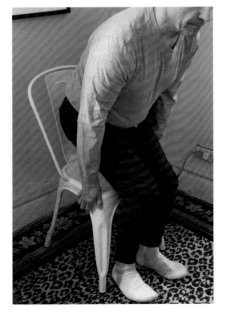

Sit to Stand

SIT TO STAND

Starting Position: Sit up tall in your chair.

Movement: Place your hands on the sides of the seat of the chair. Bend forward slightly with your back straight and look straight ahead. Now lift up out of the chair about six inches and then sit back down.

Repetitions: Repeat the movement eight times. If this is easy to do, then try extending your arms straight out in front of you as you elevate out of the chair.

Benefits: Builds strength in your gluteus muscles, which are the muscles that control sitting down and standing up. Improves overall balance.

Let's pause again and take three full breaths. Inhale slow and steady through your nose, and exhale slow and steady out your mouth.

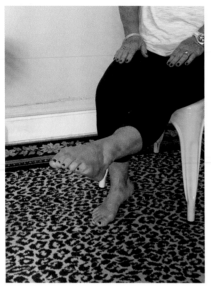

Single Leg Point and Flex

SINGLE LEG POINT AND FLEX

Starting Position: Sit tall in your chair with a straight spine.

Movement: On an inhale, extend your right leg straight out in front of you. Keeping your leg in this position, begin to point and flex your right foot. This can be done slowly or quickly. Either way, your foot and ankle get a terrific workout. Place your hands anywhere it is comfortable, whether that is down by your sides or in your lap. If possible, exaggerate both the point and the flex. When finished, return your foot to the floor and switch sides.

Repetitions: Repeat fifteen times on each side.

Benefits: Stretches shin and calf muscles while working the foot and ankle.

SINGLE LEG ANKLE CIRCLES

Starting Position: Sit tall in your chair in Mountain Pose.

Movement: Inhale as you lift your right leg up and begin to rotate your foot clockwise. Slowly articulate the circles. Make them as big and exaggerated as possible. After about ten rotations, switch direction. Keep your lifted leg as straight as possible. Switch legs.

Repetitions: Ten sets each side.

Benefits: Promotes mobility in and strengthens ankles.

Single Leg Ankle Circles

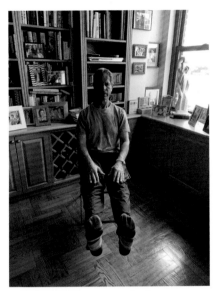
Both Legs Point and Flex

BOTH LEGS POINT AND FLEX

Starting Position: Sit in Mountain Pose.

Movement: On an inhale, extend both legs straight out in front of you. Keeping your legs in this position, begin to point and flex your feet. This can be done slowly or quickly. Either way, your feet and ankles get a terrific workout. Place your hands anywhere it is comfortable, whether that is down by your sides or in your lap. If possible, exaggerate both the point and the flex. When finished, return your feet to the floor.

Repetitions: Repeat fifteen times.

Benefits: Stretches shin and calf muscles while working the feet and ankles.

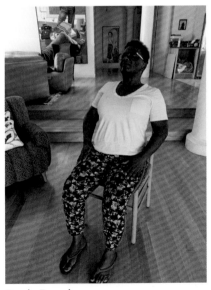
Back Bend

BACK BEND

Starting Position: Come to Mountain Pose.

Movement: Rest your hands with your palms down on your legs. On a slow, steady inhale, lift your chest, arch your back slightly, open up your shoulders, and gaze up to the ceiling. On your exhale, slowly drop your head, round your back and shoulders, and gaze down at the floor. Now return to neutral. Let's do that again. Make the four movements—lift chest, arch back, open shoulders, and gaze up—happen simultaneously on a single inhale and likewise on the exhale. This may take a bit of practice but is worth the effort.

Repetitions: Do five sets of this pose.

Benefits: Warms up the thoracic and lumbar spine (upper and lower back). Promotes good posture.

67

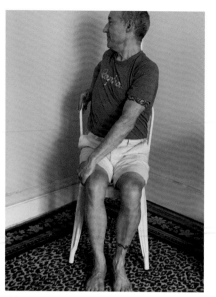

Chair Twist

CHAIR TWIST

Starting Position: Sit tall with feet hip distance apart.

Movement: Slowly twist your upper torso to your right and put your right hand on the top of the back of the chair. Place your left hand on the outside of your right knee. Make sure that both of your knees are pointing straight ahead. On an inhale, lift your spine and then exhale as you slowly twist to the right. Come back to neutral. This pose takes some practice. Do make sure that your lower body stays still!

Repetitions: Repeat five times on each side.

Benefits: Massages internal organs and tones the waistline.

Let's pause again and take three full breaths. Inhale slow and steady through your nose, and exhale slow and steady out your mouth.

EXTENDED ARMS PALM ROTATION WITH WEIGHTS

Starting Position: Shoulders back and spine straight in Mountain Pose, with weights resting in hands on your lap.

Movement: Extend both arms straight out to your sides with palms up. Weights are in each of your hands. Keep arms in extended position and rotate palms down. Switch palm position from up to down and make sure that the only part of you that is moving are your palms.

Repetitions: Do ten sets.

Benefits: Strengthens arms and warms up shoulders.

Extended Arms Palm Rotation
with Weights

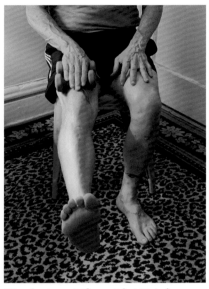

Single Leg Lifts with Weights

SINGLE LEG LIFTS WITH WEIGHTS

Starting Position: Sit tall in Mountain Pose and rest both weights on the top of your right thigh, close to your knee.

Movement: Extend your right leg out and keep it as straight as possible. Rest your right hand over the two weights and slowly begin to lift your leg up from the chair in this position. Keep your back straight as you lift.

Repetitions: Lift your straight leg ten times on each side. On the tenth rep on each side, hold the uplifted leg for one full breath. Release.

Benefits: Strengthens muscles in entire leg.

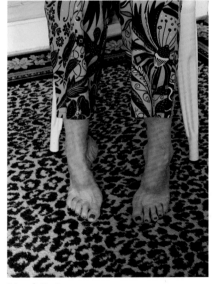

Heel Raises

HEEL RAISES

Starting Position: Sit tall and point feet straight ahead.

Movement: Keeping toes firmly planted on the floor, begin to lift your heels. Keep lifting your heels, making sure that your toes remain on the floor. If it is comfortable to do so, exaggerate the heel lift each time.

Repetitions: Repeat fifteen times.

Benefits: Stretches your calf muscles.

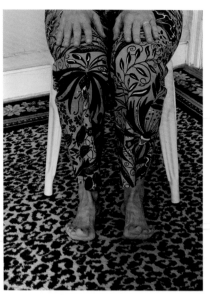

Toe Raises

TOE RAISES

Starting Position: Sit tall with feet pointed straight ahead.

   Movement: Keeping heels firmly planted on the floor, begin to lift your toes. Keep lifting your toes while making certain that your heels remain firmly on the floor. Again, if it feels okay, exaggerate the lift each time.

   Repetitions: Repeat fifteen times.

   Benefits: Stretches the shins.

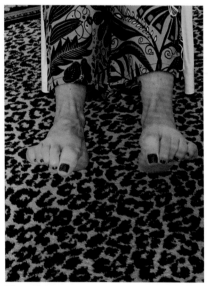

Toe Squeeze

TOE SQUEEZE/TOE SPREAD

Starting Position: Sit in Mountain Pose.

   Movement: On an inhale, extend both legs out in front. Keep them there while you begin to scrunch your toes as tightly as you can, then release the squeeze and spread your toes out as widely as possible. Scrunch again, keeping everything tight, tight, tight! Then release and spread. Imagine that you can spread your toes so wide that no toe is touching another toe. This is really just a goal to work toward. Most likely, a toe or two will be touching.

   Repetitions: Repeat this at least fifteen times. It feels good!

   Benefits: Stretches toes, feet, and ankles.

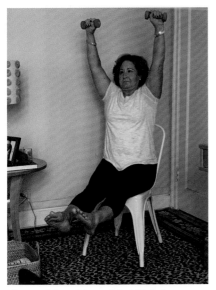

Everything Up with Weights

EVERYTHING UP WITH WEIGHTS!

Starting Position: This is your final Mountain Pose for this twenty-minute chair yoga workout. Make it a good one. Sit tall, knees hip distance apart, with toes pointing straight ahead. Keep your belly to spine. Hold weights in each hand and rest them on your legs.

Movement: On an inhale, lift your arms and legs up at the same time. Weights are in your hands. Try to keep all limbs and your back as straight as comfort will allow. Exhale, and slowly return arms and legs to starting position.

Repetitions: Repeat this pose eight times. On the last rep, hold the pose and take one full breath. Release.

Benefits: Strengthens full body.

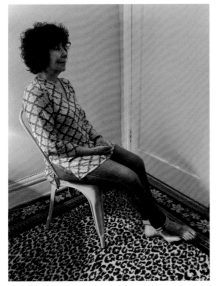

Deep Relaxation Pose

DEEP RELAXATION POSE

Starting Position: Lean back, resting your spine against the chair. Place your hands comfortably in your lap and close your eyes.

Movement: Breathe easily and relax your whole body. Allow any tension in your face, shoulders, legs, and feet to release.

Repetitions: Stay in this relaxed position for about five minutes, continuing to breathe naturally.

Benefits: Allows your body to absorb all of the benefits of your yoga practice.

Let's take three full breaths. Inhale slow and steady through your nose, and exhale slow and steady out your mouth. You have just completed a workout that, when performed three or more times a week, will change your life! Great job.

CHAPTER EIGHT

INTERMEDIATE THIRTY-MINUTE FULL BODY PROGRAM

I am so happy that you are ready to graduate to the thirty-minute intermediate routine. It is an important commitment. It will require discipline and energy. No problem, right? Let's begin with warming up.

MOUNTAIN POSE

Starting Position: Sit up nice and tall in your chair, knees comfortably hip distance apart, with toes pointed straight ahead. Place your hands on your thighs. Roll your shoulders up and then down your back and pull your navel to your spine.

THE BREATH

Starting Position: Come to sit in Mountain Pose.

  Movement: Take a slow and steady inhale through your nose, and a slow, steady exhale out your mouth. Don't force the breath. Try to

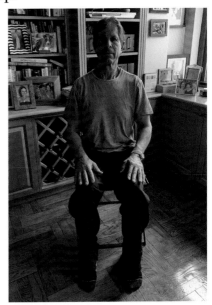

Mountain Pose

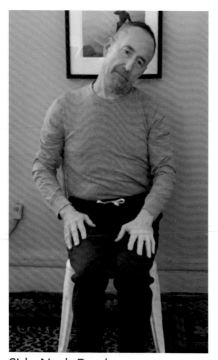

Side Neck Bend

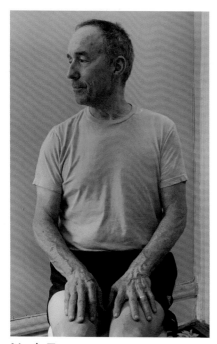

Neck Turns

make the exhale last as long as the inhale. You can start with a count of two on the inhale and a count of two on the exhale. If you can make each inhale and exhale longer, say a count of three to four, then go for it.

Repetitions: Take four complete breaths. Remember, slow and steady.

Benefits: This type of breathing calms the nervous system and reduces anxiety. It prepares your body to move.

SIDE NECK BEND

Starting Position: Come to Mountain Pose.

Movement: Inhale to sit tall. As you exhale, drop your right ear to your right shoulder. Make sure that your shoulders are relaxed. Inhale to bring your head back to neutral. Now inhale to sit tall and exhale as you bring your left ear to your left shoulder. Inhale to bring your head back to neutral. That is one set.

Repetitions: Repeat the set three times.

Benefits: Stretches the sides of the neck.

NECK TURNS

Starting Position: Return to Mountain Pose.

Movement: On an inhale, very slowly turn your head to the right. As you exhale, very slowly return to center. On an inhale, turn your head slowly to the left. On a slow and steady exhale, return to center.

Repetitions: Repeat the set three times.

Benefits: Eases tension in the neck and helps to restore mobility in the upper back.

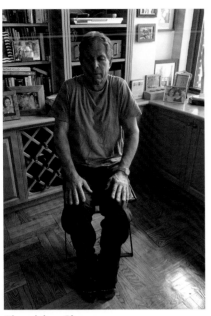

Shoulder Shrugs

SHOULDER SHRUGS

Starting Position: Resume Mountain Pose.

Movement: Inhale as you bring both shoulders up to your ears and exhale as you bring them back to neutral. Exaggerate the lift.

Repetitions: Repeat five times.

Benefits: Eases muscle tension in the neck and shoulders.

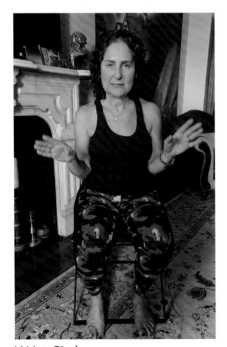

Wrist Circles

WRIST CIRCLES

Starting Position: Sit up tall in Mountain Pose. Sit with belly to spine and the crown of your head lifted toward the ceiling.

Movement: Keep your elbows close to the sides of your body and extend your hands in front of you. With fingers extended, roll your hands at the wrists. Wiggle your fingers as you roll your wrists.

Repetitions: Roll your wrists ten times, then switch direction and roll again ten times.

Benefits: Warms up the wrists and fingers. Also relieves inflammation in the hand joints.

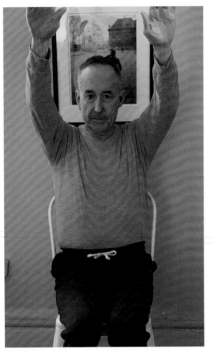

Arm Raises with Both Arms

ARM RAISES WITH BOTH ARMS

Starting Position: Assume Mountain Pose.

Movement: On a slow, steady inhale, raise both arms above your head. On a slow, steady exhale, lower your arms to starting position. Keep your shoulders relaxed during movement. If it is uncomfortable to raise your arms overhead, then raise them to a level that feels okay for you.

Repetitions: Repeat this five times.

Benefits: Encourages mobility in shoulder joints and strengthens arms.

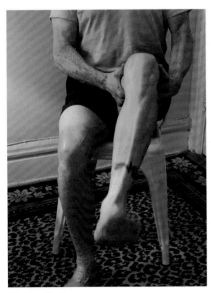

Knee Swings

KNEE SWINGS

Starting Position: Sit up tall in Mountain Pose, with belly in and shoulders back.

Movement: Clasp your hands under your right knee. Sit up tall with a straight spine. While holding under your knee, start to kick your leg out back and forth. This pose is one of the few that we do quickly. If you are unable to reach under your knee, then sit back in the chair and kick out your right leg, swinging back and forth with as much speed as is comfortable.

Repetitions: Do twenty times for each leg.

Benefits: Increases mobility and range of motion in the knees.

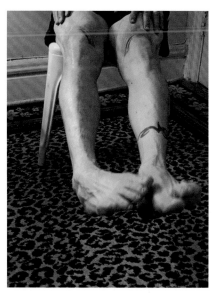

Ankle Circles with Both Legs

ANKLE CIRCLES WITH BOTH LEGS

Starting Position: Come to Mountain Pose.

Movement: On the inhale, lift your spine and extend both legs. Sit all the way back in your chair to achieve this pose. Keeping your legs as straight as you can, start to rotate your feet and ankles clockwise. The only body parts that move are your feet and ankles.

Repetitions: Rotate ten times in each direction.

Benefits: Promotes mobility in ankles and feet.

We are finished with our warm-up! Let's begin our practice.

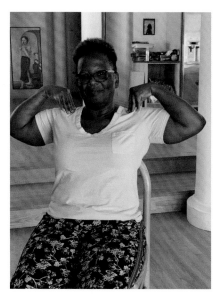

Hands on Shoulders Rolls

HANDS ON SHOULDERS ROLLS

Starting Position: Begin in Mountain Pose.

Movement: Place your hands on your shoulders and begin to make large circles with your shoulders, leading with your elbows. Breathe comfortably as you move. Switch the direction of your circles.

Repetitions: Repeat eight times in each direction.

Benefits: Warms up the upper back and releases tension in your neck.

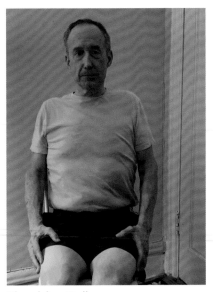

Shoulder Rolls

SHOULDER ROLLS

Starting Position: Sit up tall in Mountain Pose.

Movement: Inhale as you lift your shoulders up, then back, and exhale as you bring them around to starting position. Make the movement as smooth as possible, creating a continuous circle. After five slow and steady circles, reverse the movement. Lift your shoulders up on an inhale, bring them to the front of your body, and exhale as you bring your shoulders back to starting position. This direction always feels awkward. Don't worry, you are doing it correctly!

Repetitions: Repeat the movement eight times in each direction.

Benefits: Opens up the shoulder joints and improves mobility.

FORWARD BEND WITH STRAIGHT BACK

Starting Position: Sit up tall in your chair with palms resting on your thighs.

Movement: On an inhale, bend forward from the hips, leading with your chin. Keep your spine straight. Go only as far as you can with your back straight. The bend is from the hips. On the exhale, come back up using your hands on your legs to push you back up. Look straight ahead throughout the movement. Do not look down. Depending on your spine's flexibility,

Forward Bend with Straight Back

78

this movement may be small. That is absolutely okay. Remember, the movement is slow!

Repetitions: Repeat eight times. On the eighth rep, hold the bent position and take one full breath consisting of a slow, steady inhale and a slow, steady exhale. Return to neutral.

Benefits: Expands mobility in the back and strengthens the muscles of the lower back.

ALTERNATING ARM RAISES WITH WEIGHTS

Starting Position: Come to Mountain Pose holding the two-pound weights in your hands as they rest on your thighs.

Movement: Inhale as you lift your right arm above your head, only if this movement is pain free. If it isn't, then lift your arm as high as it will go comfortably. Try to keep your extended arm straight and your shoulder relaxed. Exhale as you lower your arm down. Switch sides.

Repetitions: Repeat six times on each side. Hold the pose on the last rep of each side and take two full breaths. Release pose and return to neutral. You are holding the weights in both hands throughout the exercise.

Benefits: Lubricates the shoulder joint and strengthens the arms.

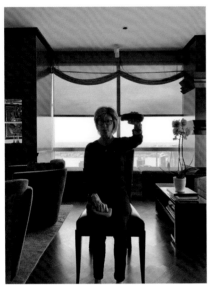

Alternating Arm Raises with Weights

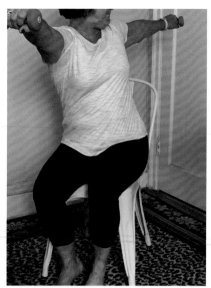

Torso Twist with Arms Extended with Weights

TORSO TWIST WITH ARMS EXTENDED WITH WEIGHTS

Starting Position: Assume the Mountain Pose with weights in each hand.

Movement: Hold a weight in each hand and on an inhale, extend your arms out to the sides. Exhale. On an inhale, twist slowly to your right. Your head travels with your extended right arm. Exhale back to neutral. Don't lower your arms. If you are using a mirror, check to see that your extended arms are even and that your shoulders are down. Inhale and twist to your left. Your head travels with your left arm. Return to neutral and bring your arms down with hands resting on your legs.

Repetitions: Repeat each set eight times. Hold the pose on the last rep on each side and take two full breaths. Release pose and return to neutral.

Benefits: Tones waistline and strengthens arms.

Let's pause and take three full breaths. Inhale slow and steady through your nose, and exhale slow and steady out your mouth.

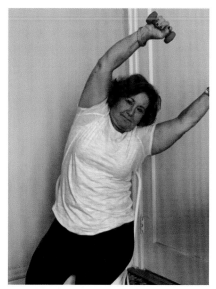

Side Body Lean with Weights

SIDE BODY LEAN WITH WEIGHTS

Starting Position: Sit up nice and tall in Mountain Pose. Take weights in each hand and rest them on your thighs.

Movement: With weights in both hands, inhale as you lift both arms up and stay. Exhale. On your next inhale, lean to your right. Exhale as you lift your arms back up to neutral. On a slow, steady inhale, with arms still up over your head, lean to your left. Exhale as you lift both arms back up overhead.

Repetitions: Do eight sets. Arms stay up throughout. On the last rep on each side, hold the pose and take two full breaths. Release pose and return to neutral.

Benefits: Tones waistline.

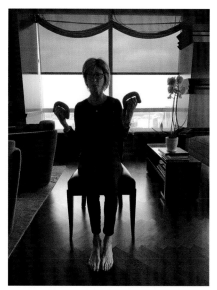

Bicep Curls Alternating Arms with Weights

BICEP CURLS ALTERNATING ARMS WITH WEIGHTS

Starting Position: Come to sit in Mountain Pose with the weights in your hands.

Movement: Drop your arms by your sides. Keep your elbows glued to the sides of your body. On the inhale, slowly bend your right arm up and exhale as you lower it down to starting position. Inhale as you bring the left arm up and exhale to bring it back to start. Your elbows never leave the sides of your torso during the movement.

Repetitions: Repeat eight times on each side. Pause for a breath and repeat the exercise for eight reps on each side.

Benefits: Builds muscle in the biceps.

81

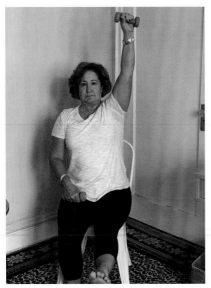

Single Arm and Leg Raises with Weights

SINGLE ARM AND LEG RAISES WITH WEIGHTS

Starting Position: Come to Mountain Pose with weights resting in your lap.

Movement: Inhale as you lift your right arm (weight is in your hand) and right leg together. Both your arm and leg should be as straight as you can make them. Exhale as you lower them.

Repetitions: Repeat six times on each side. Hold pose in the up position on the last rep of each side and take two full breaths. Release the pose and return to neutral.

Benefits: Strengthens arm and leg muscles. Expands coordination.

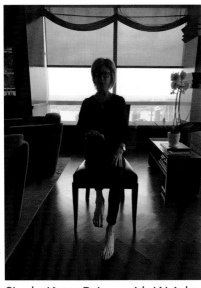

Single Knee Raises with Weights

SINGLE KNEE RAISES WITH WEIGHTS

Starting Position: Sit up tall in Mountain Pose with both weights resting on the top of your right knee.

Movement: Resting your right hand over the two weights to hold them in place, slowly lift your right knee straight up and then slowly lower your foot to the floor. Repeat ten times. On the final rep, hold your knee up and take two full breaths. Return your foot to the floor and switch sides. Place the two weights on top of your left knee.

Repetitions: Repeat ten times on each side. Hold your knee in up position and take two full breaths on the last rep of each side. Release pose.

Benefits: Strengthens quadriceps.

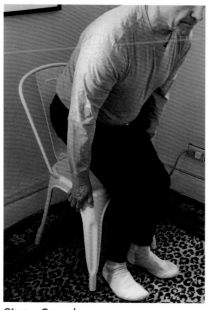

Sit to Stand

SIT TO STAND

Starting Position: Sit up tall in your chair.

Movement: Place your hands on the sides of the seat of the chair. Bend forward slightly with your back straight and look straight ahead. Now lift up out of the chair about six inches and then sit back down.

Repetitions: Repeat the movement eight times. If this is easy to do, then try extending your arms straight out in front of you as you elevate out of the chair.

Benefits: Builds strength in your gluteus muscles, which are the muscles that control sitting down and standing up. Improves overall balance.

Let's pause again and take three full breaths. Inhale slow and steady through your nose, and exhale slow and steady out your mouth.

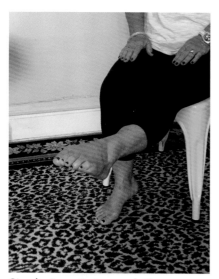

Single Leg Point and Flex

SINGLE LEG POINT AND FLEX

Starting Position: Sit tall in your chair with a straight spine.

Movement: On an inhale, extend your right leg straight out in front of you. Keeping your leg in this position, begin to point and flex your right foot. This can be done slowly or quickly. Either way, your foot and ankle get a terrific workout. Place your hands anywhere it is comfortable, whether that is down by your sides or in your lap. If possible, exaggerate both the point and the flex. When finished, return your foot to the floor and switch sides.

Repetitions: Repeat fifteen times on each side.

Benefits: Stretches shin and calf muscles while working the foot and ankle.

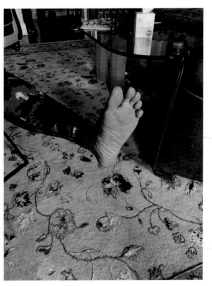

Single Leg Ankle Circles

SINGLE LEG ANKLE CIRCLES

Starting Position: Sit tall in your chair in Mountain Pose.

Movement: Inhale as you lift your right leg up and begin to rotate your foot clockwise. Slowly articulate the circles. Make them as big and exaggerated as possible. After about ten rotations, switch direction. Keep your lifted leg as straight as possible. Switch legs.

Repetitions: Ten sets each side.

Benefits: Promotes mobility in and strengthens ankles.

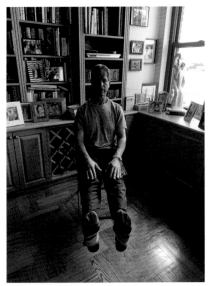

Both Legs Point and Flex

BOTH LEGS POINT AND FLEX

Starting Position: Sit in Mountain Pose.

Movement: On an inhale, extend both legs straight out in front of you. Keeping your legs in this position, begin to point and flex your feet. This can be done slowly or quickly. Either way, your feet and ankles get a terrific workout. Place your hands anywhere it is comfortable, whether that is down by your sides or in your lap. If possible, exaggerate both the point and the flex. When finished, return your feet to the floor.

Repetitions: Repeat fifteen times.

Benefits: Stretches shin and calf muscles while working the feet and ankles.

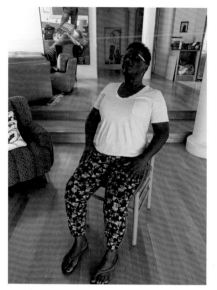
Back Bend

BACK BEND

Starting Position: Come to Mountain Pose.

Movement: Rest your hands with your palms down on your legs. On a slow, steady inhale, lift your chest, arch your back slightly, open up your shoulders, and gaze up to the ceiling. On your exhale, slowly drop your head, round your back and shoulders, and gaze down at the floor. Now return to neutral. Let's do that again. Make the four movements—lift chest, arch back, open shoulders, and gaze up—happen simultaneously on a single inhale and likewise on the exhale. This may take a bit of practice but is worth the effort.

Repetitions: Do five sets of this pose.

Benefits: Warms up the thoracic and lumbar spine (upper and lower back). Promotes good posture.

CHAIR TWIST

Starting Position: Sit tall with feet hip distance apart.

Movement: Slowly twist your upper torso to your right and put your right hand on the top of the back of the chair. Place your left hand on the outside of your right knee. Make sure that both of your knees are pointing straight ahead. On an inhale, lift your spine and then exhale as you slowly twist to the right. Come back to neutral. This pose takes some practice. Do make sure that your lower body stays still!

Repetitions: Repeat five times on each side.

Benefits: Massages internal organs and tones the waistline.

Chair Twist

85

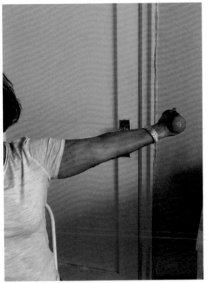

Extended Arms Palm Rotation
with Weights

EXTENDED ARMS PALM ROTATION WITH WEIGHTS

Starting Position: Shoulders back and spine straight in Mountain Pose, with weights resting in hands on your lap.

Movement: Extend both arms straight out to your sides with palms up. Weights are in each of your hands. Keep arms in extended position and rotate palms down. Switch palm position from up to down and make sure that the only part of you that is moving are your palms.

Repetitions: Do ten sets.

Benefits: Strengthens arms and warms up shoulders.

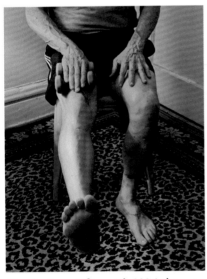

Single Leg Lifts with Weights

SINGLE LEG LIFTS WITH WEIGHTS

Starting Position: Sit tall in Mountain Pose and rest both weights on the top of your right thigh close to your knee.

Movement: Extend your right leg out and keep it as straight as possible. Rest your right hand over the two weights and slowly begin to lift your leg up from the chair in this position. Keep your back straight as you lift.

Repetitions: Lift your straight leg eight times on each side. On the eighth rep on each side, hold the uplifted leg for two full breaths. Release.

Benefits: Strengthens muscles in entire leg.

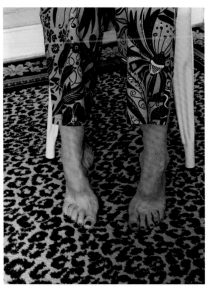

Heel Raises

HEEL RAISES

Starting Position: Sit tall and point feet straight ahead.

Movement: Keeping toes firmly planted on the floor, begin to lift your heels. Keep lifting your heels, making sure that your toes remain on the floor. If it is comfortable to do so, exaggerate the heel lift each time.

Repetitions: Repeat fifteen times.

Benefits: Stretches your calf muscles.

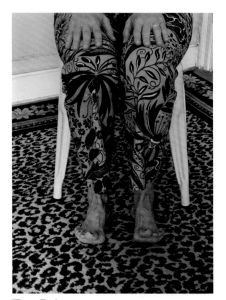

Toe Raises

TOE RAISES

Starting Position: Sit tall with feet pointed straight ahead.

Movement: Keeping heels firmly planted on the floor, begin to lift your toes. Keep lifting your toes while making certain that your heels remain firmly on the floor. Again, if it feels okay, exaggerate the lift each time.

Repetitions: Repeat fifteen times.

Benefits: Stretches the shins.

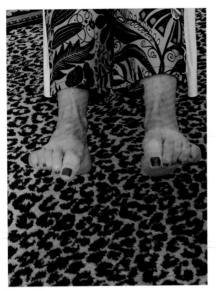

Toe Squeeze

TOE SQUEEZE/TOE SPREAD

Starting Position: Sit in Mountain Pose.

Movement: On an inhale, extend both legs out in front. Keep them there while you begin to scrunch your toes as tightly as you can, then release the squeeze and spread your toes out as widely as possible. Scrunch again, keeping everything tight, tight, tight! Then release and spread. Imagine that you can spread your toes so wide that no toe is touching another toe. This is really just a goal to work toward. Most likely, a toe or two will be touching.

Repetitions: Repeat this at least fifteen times. It feels good!

Benefits: Stretches toes, feet, and ankles.

EVERYTHING UP WITH WEIGHTS!

Starting Position: This is your final Mountain Pose for this thirty-minute chair yoga workout. Make it a good one. Sit tall, knees hip distance apart, with toes pointing straight ahead. Keep your belly to spine. Hold weights in each hand and rest them on your legs.

Movement: On an inhale, lift your arms and legs up at the same time. Weights are in your hands. Try to keep all limbs and your back as straight as comfort will allow. Exhale, and slowly return arms and legs to starting position.

Repetitions: Repeat this pose eight times. On the last rep, hold the pose and take two full breaths. Release.

Everything Up with Weights

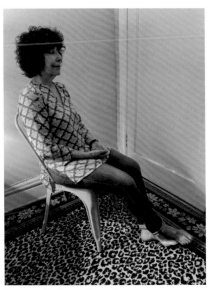

Deep Relaxation Pose

Benefits: Strengthens full body.

DEEP RELAXATION POSE

Starting Position: Lean back, resting your spine against the chair. Place your hands comfortably in your lap and close your eyes.

Movement: Breathe easily and relax your whole body. Allow any tension in your face, shoulders, legs, and feet to release.

Repetitions: Stay in this relaxed position for about five minutes, continuing to breathe naturally.

Benefits: Allows your body to absorb all of the benefits of your yoga practice.

Take three full breaths. Inhale slow and steady through your nose, and exhale slow and steady out your mouth.

This is a major achievement. You completed thirty minutes of a rigorous chair yoga routine. The challenging part is to commit to it at least three times a week. This constitutes a habit! A very good, healthy habit.

CHAPTER NINE

YOU CAN DO THIS ANYWHERE!

Once your exercise habit kicks in, I believe you will embrace the realization that, next to being with family and friends, routine exercise is the most important thing that you can do for yourself. Consistent exercise puts you on the path to a more positive outlook on life, and reduces anxiety and pain.

The next logical extension of this new part of your life is the realization that you can do most of these exercises anywhere. Really, you can complete the exercises listed in this book almost anywhere.

Let me help you think this through. If you are sitting in a chair at a friend's home, in a doctor's waiting room, on an airplane, on a bus, or as a passenger in a car; you can be moving your body in beneficial ways. Obviously, you don't want to attract any unwanted attention, so below I list the poses that you can do in subtle ways that will add to the level of fitness that you worked so hard to achieve.

The very first pose that you learned here—in many ways the most important one of all the poses listed here—is Mountain Pose. Even if you are sitting on a couch or a cushy chair, you can sit up tall and straight, pulling your belly in, lifting and opening your shoulders, keeping your knees and feet pointed straight ahead, and breathing in a slow and steady flow. If you are sitting for an extended period of time, you can keep coming back to this position and method of breathing.

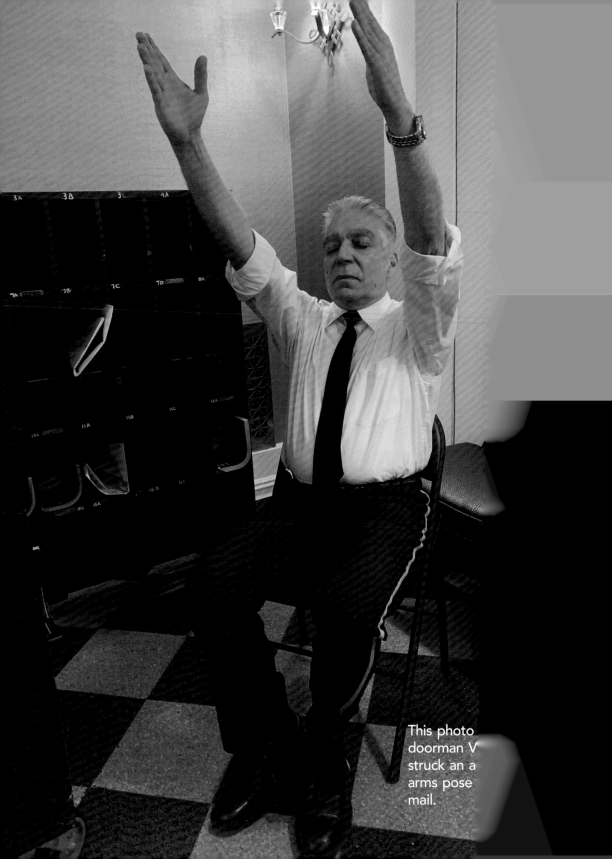

This photo
doorman V
struck an a
arms pose
mail.

Moving on from Mountain Pose, let's try to keep our neck free from stress and tension. We can do that by utilizing slow and steady neck turns and side neck bends. This is the ear to shoulder movement from our warm-up routine.

Moving down the list of poses from the beginner series, let's loosen up our shoulders by doing a few shoulder rolls.

The next pose, one that always feels good, is the forward bend with straight back. Do this a few times using a slow and steady breath to experience a gentle spine stretch.

Let's move on to the lower body. If there is room in front of you—maybe not in a car or on a plane, but likely anyplace—do some single leg raises. This will aid circulation in your lower extremities. Another pose that is easy to do from any sitting location is knee raises. It strengthens the muscles surrounding the knee joint.

Last, but never least, are the poses for the feet. We can do all of them in an unobtrusive way.

Try a single leg point and flex, and a single leg ankle circle. If you aren't comfortable sticking your leg straight out to do these, you can lift your foot up a few inches from the floor and proceed.

Finally, there heel and toe raises, which are so beneficial to foot health, and can easily be done anywhere you take a seat.

What if you are alone, in your home watching TV or just relaxing with a book or magazine?

Try toe squeezes, wrist circles, both legs ankle circles, both legs point and flex, alternating arm raises, and knee swings. You can do any or all of the poses. Go in order. Go out of order. Do three poses. Just make sure to breathe mindfully. Take three slow and steady inhales and exhales. Do ten poses. Just do toe squeezes.

Are you getting my point? Anywhere you are, whatever you are doing, try to move your body parts. Lengthen, extend, and expand your muscles and joints in the ways you have learned in this book. These are the tools you have acquired to achieve and maintain a healthy body and healthy mind.

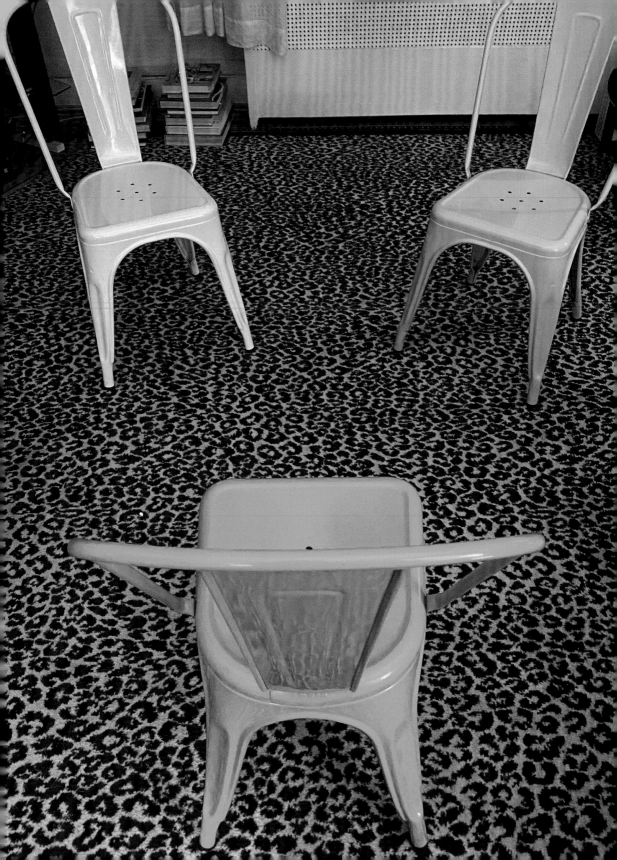

CHAPTER TEN

INVITE FRIENDS TO JOIN YOU

Have you been practicing chair yoga regularly for a few months now and can't stop talking about it to anyone who will listen? I'm guessing yes and I'm also guessing that it is partly due to the compliments you have been getting. A regular exercise habit shows in our face, on our body, in how we walk, and in how we communicate with others. It allows us to feel calmer and less stressed. It clears our mind, especially when we do mindful breathing on a regular basis.

I'm sure you have noticed that I use the word "habit" a lot. This isn't accidental. A habit is something you do regularly without thinking too much about it. You are automatically driven to do it. A habit isn't something you do occasionally. A habit can be good, or it can be bad. Most likely, the bad habit that comes to mind first for most of us is smoking. Some really good habits are exercise, reading, and volunteering. I'm sure that you can think of many more.

The key to the habit is consistency. A chair yoga practice of at least three times a week is a habit. In addition to this, you can do a few extra poses throughout the day wherever you may be sitting. Consistency is the key.

Now what does this have to do with sharing with friends? If you have developed the habit of exercise and acknowledge the benefits, you will naturally want to share your experience with friends. By share I mean more than just telling them about your experience and encouraging them to give it a try. I am suggesting forming a small group and doing it together in your home or anyone else's. How do you do it? Here are some suggestions.

Find a space big enough to accommodate a few chairs. I would begin this group adventure with one or two friends and if successful, you can expand. Set up the chairs in a horseshoe format. This layout allows for eye contact with each other. Make sure that when everyone is seated that each person can extend their arms and legs in all directions without hitting each other.

Ideally, each participant should have a *Chair Yoga for Seniors* book. If not, whoever has the book will be reading the instructions. Since you have been doing this for a while, you could probably recite the instructions from memory. Do resist doing this, however, since your friends, who you have invited over, will need to hear all of the minute details to execute the poses properly.

Agree upon the music you will listen to. Chances are you will have similar music tastes as your friends. Be creative here. If anyone in your group is a user of Spotify or Apple Music, they can create a fun playlist for your group sessions.

This should be a fun endeavor. Establish a few ground rules but go easy on each other. Don't worry about timing. Take as much time as everyone needs to understand how to do each pose correctly. Since you, my reader, brought this group together, remind everyone to work within their own range of mobility and to not do any exercise that causes pain.

Now everyone, drink a glass of water and begin the warm-ups!

CHAPTER ELEVEN

I FEEL SO MUCH BETTER. I WANT MORE!

I'm sure that friends and family have noticed some of the changes in you since you began practicing chair yoga regularly. You are standing taller, have more confidence in your step, have a brighter outlook on life, and are breathing easier. I hope that this has made you hungry for more. More what? I will tell you. There are so many lifestyle changes and enhancements that are available to us to make our lives happier, healthier, and more fulfilling. If you are ready to open up yourself and your life to having more health, happiness, fulfillment, purpose, and serenity, then stay with me for the this chapter. I want to share some of the joys of my journey that can help you expand your horizons.

If you are prepared to explore, then I must ask you to bear with me as I make a few assumptions about you. I imagine that you bought this book with the intention of trying something that would make you feel better. You probably started with the beginner programs and gained the confidence and strength to move on to the intermediate section of the book. By now a chair yoga routine is a part of your daily life. Not only do you set up your home space to work through a twenty- or thirty-minute program three or more times a week, you can move your neck, shoulders, legs, and feet wherever you find yourself seated. You feel good. Better than you have in a long time. You have less tension and stress and your aches and pains are more controlled. Am I describing you? Or some version of you? If you can relate to any of the details I have just listed, then you are ready to open up your mind, heart, and body to experience a truly holistic, healthy life.

I am going to cover four pursuits that have been well-documented for their effectiveness and will contribute in significant ways to the betterment of your life. I will then move on with a thirty-minute advanced chair yoga/weight training routine, if you feel ready to try.

The four areas we will explore are:

- The advantages of healthy eating.
- The benefits of meditation.
- The rewards of volunteering.
- The power of community and social connection.

HEALTHY EATING

Let's start with having a healthy diet. There are so many weight loss schemes that are touted throughout the media. Often it is hard to tell the difference between commercials and content. There are meal plans that are delivered to you, additional protein drinks and supplements, guidelines for when to eat, when to fast, etc. It is dizzying! I grew up in a traditional Italian-American household where food was in abundance. We encouraged each other to eat! Eating was a social experience. So much focus on food. It took me decades to reduce the importance of food in my life. I am still working at it. I do maintain a healthy weight. However, it isn't easy for me. Over the years when I would find the scale creeping upwards, I would try a variety of weight loss methods. What worked for me was maintaining a healthy diet.

What is a healthy diet? There are few diets as universally recommended by experts as the Mediterranean diet. It really is more of a lifestyle than a diet. It

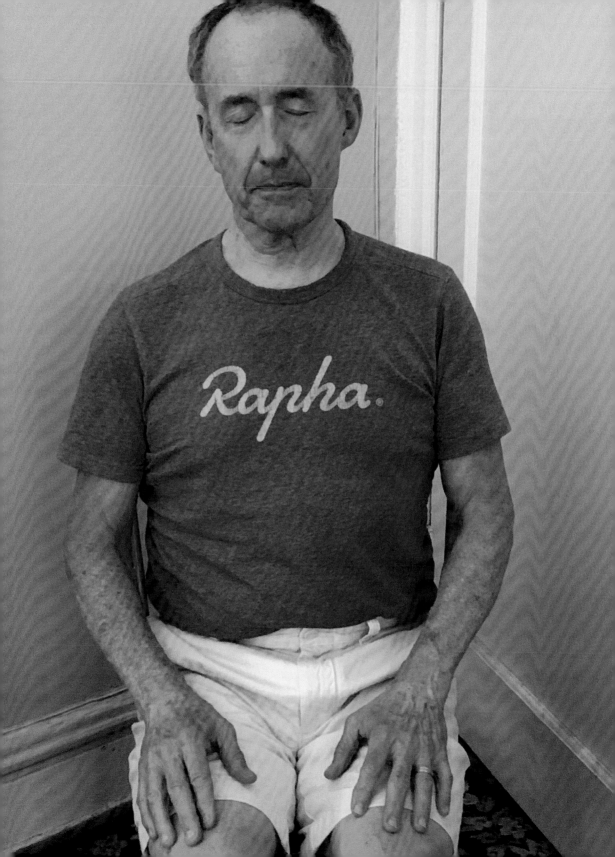

is linked to twenty-five percent lower risk for heart disease. It is also routinely recommended to people with type 2 diabetes.

What does a Mediterranean diet consist of? It is a plant-based diet with protein as a "side." That means lots of vegetables and fruit, limited skinless chicken and fish, and moderate amounts of beans, nuts, and healthy fats such as olive oil and avocados. Limited amounts of sweets and alcohol are allowed. Are you wondering about bread and pasta? I know that you are. Whole grains! This is a must. Any bread that you eat should be made with whole grains. Check the packaging. Wheat flour is not the same as whole wheat. Make sure that the word whole is used to describe the grain. This also is for pasta. Whole wheat pasta is delicious and readily available in stores and on menus.

If you are looking to drop a few pounds, then go easy on the whole grain bread and pasta and the nuts. All are high in calories.

A wonderful resource for information on how to follow the Mediterranean diet is Oldwayspt.org. In 1993, Oldways created the Mediterranean Diet Pyramid in partnership with the Harvard School of Public Health and the World Health Organization (WHO) as a healthier alternative to the USDA's original food pyramid. It has all the information you need to understand how and why to pursue this as a lifestyle.

MEDITATION

If you haven't ever meditated, you are likely to dismiss it as some new-age endeavor that isn't for you. I would like to debunk any myths you may believe about meditation and introduce you to something that will have a positive impact on your ability to handle stress and feel peaceful, while lowering your blood pressure and heart rate! I know, it sounds too good to be true. But it is true.

Meditation in its simplest form is about giving your brain a rest from all of the many thoughts that are racing through your mind every waking hour. It is simple to do and can be effective when practiced for as little as five minutes a day. Like an exercise habit, meditation is best when it is done regularly. Devoting five to ten minutes a day to a meditation practice will allow you to reduce the stress of the many challenges we all face as we age and channel it away from depression and insomnia.

How do you do it? First, find a comfortable spot to sit where your back is supported and you feel relaxed. Uncross your legs and arms and place your hands in your lap. When you are first getting accustomed to a meditation habit, you may want to use some form of a timer. A kitchen timer, a stop watch, or any gadget that you can set for five or more minutes will work well.

Allow your body and mind to unwind. Start with your eyes open, but keep your focus soft. Take a few big breaths and then gently close your eyes. Breathe naturally. Focus your attention on how your body feels. Start at your head and scan down your body. Gently breathe. Feel how your belly expands on the inhale and your shoulders relax on the exhale. Don't worry if thoughts come across your mind. Gently bring your attention back to your breath. You can think about the air filling your body on the inhale and leaving your body on the exhale. You can also think the words *I am breathing in, I am breathing out.* This will center you and bring you back to your meditation. When the time is up, open your eyes slowly and take in the room.

Many people find it is easier to stick to a meditation habit if they do it the same time every day. If this isn't practical for you then do it anytime you can set aside a quiet five to ten minutes.

If you would like to experiment with different types of meditation I encourage you to check out the Headspace App that is available on your smartphone, or look for guided meditations on YouTube. A great time to meditate is immediately following your chair yoga practice. You created the perfect setting for your exercise. It is a very easy transition.

VOLUNTEERING

Volunteering is the most selfish thing you can do. Yes, you read that correctly. What could I possibly mean by that? I will explain. Usually when we decide to volunteer for something, we are thinking in terms of helping a person, a cause, a movement, or an organization. We would be absolutely right in our assumption. To help anyone without having to do it or getting paid is usually greatly appreciated. Volunteering also has important emotional and physical health benefits for the volunteer—especially when that volunteer is a senior. According to the National Institute on Aging, participating in meaningful social activities, like volunteering, can improve longevity, boost mental health, and reduce the risk of dementia. To cite another study, one conducted by the Corporation for National and Community Service, adults over the age of sixty who volunteer reported higher levels of overall well-being than those who did not volunteer. Bottom line, we get so much more out of the act of volunteering than those who are the beneficiaries of our efforts.

I believe that the secret to a truly rewarding volunteer experience is to find something that is personally meaningful. If you have a particular talent, expertise, or passion, the chance to share it or teach it to others is one of the paths to a purpose-driven life. As I reflect on this I call to mind a handful of examples of people who have reaped the benefits of volunteering.

Sandy is in her late sixties and retired. She was a French major in college and loves all things French. Once a week she teaches French to a group of seniors at a community center. She loves sharing her passion and gets very excited when individuals in her group make breakthroughs.

Greg, a retired lawyer, volunteers once a week at New York City's Legal Aid Society. He is so happy when he counsels someone in need.

Fred, a retired business owner, volunteers his time to an organization called SCORE. It is the nation's largest network of volunteer, expert business mentors helping those who want to start businesses of their own. Fred was very successful and is gratified to pay it forward.

Are you wondering what my volunteer routine is? I thought you'd never ask. Every Friday I teach chair yoga to an Alzheimer's group at an adult day-care center. I have been doing it for four years and never tire of the joy I feel when I can get a group of people, who do not move nearly enough, to follow my direction and experience all of the benefits of exercise.

My most touching volunteer story is about my Uncle Bill, who passed at the age of ninety-six. Up until two weeks before he died, he spent two days a week as a volunteer at the VA hospital in Seminole, Florida. He had done this for the past twenty years. Bill was a WWII veteran and was profoundly affected by the experience. He was driven by the need to help veterans injured in all of the wars that came after the "big one." Nothing could keep Bill from his two-day a week commitment. He battled cancer numerous times and kept up his visits to the VA throughout treatment. He was my shining example of giving back, paying it forward, and experiencing the power of humanity.

COMMUNITY AND SOCIAL CONNECTION

According to researcher Sheldon Cohen of Carnegie Mellon University, there are two essential aspects of our social worlds that contribute to health: social support and social integration. I will focus here on the integration aspect of community connection. As we enter our senior years, our day-to-day life changes in dramatic ways. Children are grown and long gone from our homes. We are likely to be retired and no longer connect with colleagues on a daily basis. Our routines, ones that we had for decades, cease to exist. Some welcome this newfound "freedom" from work and family, but many more are basically in mourning for a past life that was filled with purpose and obligation. Unless we create a new way to live happily, we are prone to depression, weight gain, and failing health. Many of you who are reading this book have successfully transitioned and have strong social and community support. I'm sure that you could help me with examples of the healing power of community. For those of you who have struggled with finding the community activity that speaks to you and your interests, I want to help you get started.

An important community opportunity is joining an exercise class. Silver Sneakers is an ideal program for seniors. It is available all over the country and is usually a benefit of Medicare or Medicare's supplemental insurance. The classes are typically joined by the same group of people who bond before, during, and after the class. My ninety-four-year old mother attends a Silver Sneakers class three times a week in Largo, Florida. Her fellow classmates help her set up her chair and dumbbells. On her ninety-fourth birthday, the teacher brought in a cake for the class to celebrate. That is community!

There are so many ways to join groups. I belong to a reading group and a knitting circle. I love to read and knit, but meeting with my two groups brings me so much more joy than getting books read and sweaters knitted. I love and thrive on the social connection.

Think of people who golf. Strong social connections are made. Card games such as Bridge and Poker are activities where players meet regularly, sharing a love of the game.

What if you aren't a "joiner" by nature? Well, maybe it's time to give it a try. Take a class at a local college. Learn a new language. Learn to play an instrument. Do you play pool? Bowl? Join a league. Find something! Find more than one thing. It will make you feel better, stronger, and more supported.

CHAPTER TWELVE

ADVANCED THIRTY-MINUTE FULL BODY PROGRAM

The only additional equipment you will need for this routine are a set each of three- and four-pound weights. In this routine, there is a greater focus on building and maintaining muscle strength than in the beginner and intermediate programs. Always modify as you see fit. At this point in your yoga habit, you are more in touch with what your body can and cannot handle. Listen to it.

Begin this routine, as you always do, by doing five minutes of warm-ups.

Once your warm-up is complete, you can begin. Keep both the three- and four-pound weights close by. Don't forget to drink water before and after.

MOUNTAIN POSE

Starting Position: Sit up nice and tall in your chair, knees comfortably hip distance apart,

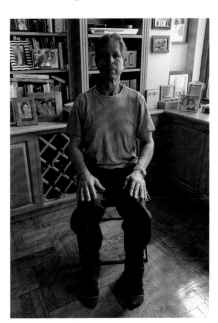

Mountain Pose

with toes pointed straight ahead. Place your hands on your thighs. Roll your shoulders up and then down your back and pull your navel to your spine.

THE BREATH

Starting Position: Come to sit in Mountain Pose.

Movement: Take a slow and steady inhale through your nose, and a slow, steady exhale out your mouth. Don't force the breath. Try to make the exhale last as long as the inhale. You can start with a count of two on the inhale and a count of two on the exhale. If you can make each inhale and exhale longer, say a count of three to four, then go for it.

Repetitions: Take four complete breaths. Remember, slow and steady.

Benefits: This type of breathing calms the nervous system and reduces anxiety. It prepares your body to move.

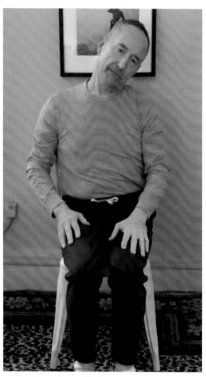

Side Neck Bend

SIDE NECK BEND

Starting Position: Come to Mountain Pose.

Movement: Inhale to sit tall. As you exhale, drop your right ear to your right shoulder. Make sure that your shoulders are relaxed. Inhale to bring your head back to neutral. Now inhale to sit tall and exhale as you bring your left ear to your left shoulder. Inhale to bring your head back to neutral. That is one set.

Repetitions: Repeat the set three times.

Benefits: Stretches the sides of the neck.

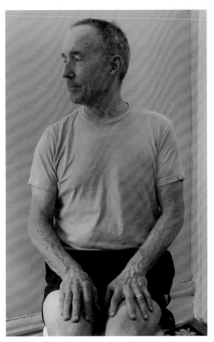

Neck Turns

NECK TURNS

Starting Position: Return to Mountain Pose.

Movement: On an inhale, very slowly turn your head to the right. As you exhale, very slowly return to center. On an inhale, turn your head slowly to the left. On a slow and steady exhale, return to center.

Repetitions: Repeat the set three times.

Benefits: Eases tension in the neck and helps to restore mobility in the upper back.

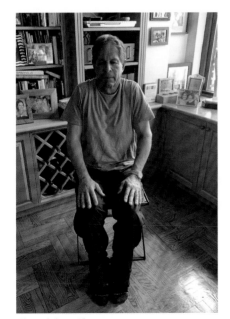

Shoulder Shrugs

SHOULDER SHRUGS

Starting Position: Resume Mountain Pose.

Movement: Inhale as you bring both shoulders up to your ears and exhale as you bring them back to neutral. Exaggerate the lift.

Repetitions: Repeat five times.

Benefits: Eases muscle tension in the neck and shoulders.

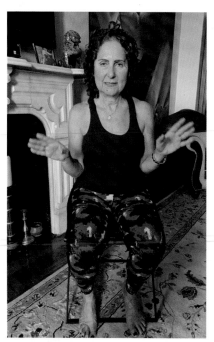

Wrist Circles

WRIST CIRCLES

Starting Position: Sit up tall in Mountain Pose. Sit with belly to spine and the crown of your head lifted toward the ceiling.

Movement: Keep your elbows close to the sides of your body and extend your hands in front of you. With fingers extended, roll your hands at the wrists. Wiggle your fingers as you roll your wrists.

Repetitions: Roll your wrists ten times, then switch direction and roll again ten times.

Benefits: Warms up the wrists and fingers. Also relieves inflammation in the hand joints.

ARM RAISES WITH BOTH ARMS

Starting Position: Assume Mountain Pose.

Movement: On a slow, steady inhale, raise both arms above your head. On a slow, steady exhale, lower your arms to starting position. Keep your shoulders relaxed during movement. If it is uncomfortable to raise your arms overhead, then raise them to a level that feels okay for you.

Repetitions: Repeat this five times.

Benefits: Encourages mobility in shoulder joints and strengthens arms.

Arm Raises with Both Arms

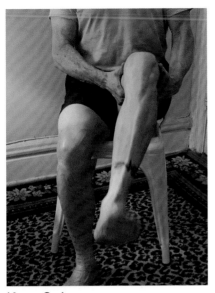
Knee Swings

KNEE SWINGS

Starting Position: Sit up tall in Mountain Pose, with belly in and shoulders back.

Movement: Clasp your hands under your right knee. Sit up tall with a straight spine. While holding under your knee, start to kick your leg out back and forth. This pose is one of the few that we do quickly. If you are unable to reach under your knee, then sit back in the chair and kick out your right leg, swinging back and forth with as much speed as is comfortable.

Repetitions: Do twenty times for each leg.

Benefits: Increases mobility and range of motion in the knees.

ANKLE CIRCLES WITH BOTH LEGS

Starting Position: Come to Mountain Pose.

Movement: On the inhale, lift your spine and extend both legs. Sit all the way back in your chair to achieve this pose. Keeping your legs as straight as you can, start to rotate your feet and ankles clockwise. The only body parts that move are your feet and ankles.

Repetitions: Rotate ten times in each direction.

Benefits: Promotes mobility in ankles and feet.

Ankle Circles with Both Legs

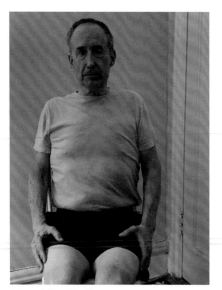

Shoulder Rolls

SHOULDER ROLLS

Starting Position: Sit up tall in Mountain Pose.

Movement: Inhale as you lift your shoulders up, then back, and exhale as you bring them around to starting position. Make the movement as smooth as possible, creating a continuous circle. After five slow and steady circles, reverse the movement. Lift your shoulders up on an inhale, bring them to the front of your body, and exhale as you bring your shoulders back to starting position. This direction always feels awkward. Don't worry, you are doing it correctly!

Repetitions: Repeat the movement eight times in each direction.

Benefits: Opens up the shoulder joints and improves mobility.

Shoulder Rolls with Weights

SHOULDER ROLLS WITH WEIGHTS

Starting Position: Sit up tall in Mountain Pose with a weight in each hand.

Movement: Inhale as you lift your shoulders up, then back, and exhale as you bring them around to starting position. Make the movement as smooth as possible, creating a continuous circle. After five slow and steady circles, reverse the movement. Lift your shoulders up on an inhale, bring them to the front of your body, and exhale as you bring your shoulders back to starting position. This direction feels awkward for everyone. Don't worry, you are doing it correctly!

Repetitions: Repeat the movement eight times in each direction.

Benefits: Opens up the shoulder joints and improves mobility.

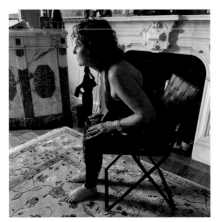

Forward Bend with Straight Back

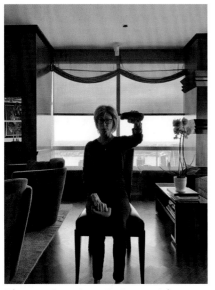

Alternating Arm Raises with Weights

FORWARD BEND WITH STRAIGHT BACK

Starting Position: Sit up tall in your chair with palms resting on your thighs.

Movement: On an inhale, bend forward from the hips, leading with your chin. Keep your spine straight. Go only as far as you can with your back straight. The bend is from the hips. On the exhale, come back up using your hands on your legs to push you back up. Look straight ahead throughout the movement. Do not look down. Depending on your spine's flexibility, this movement may be small. That is absolutely okay. Remember, the movement is slow!

Repetitions: Repeat eight times. On the eighth rep, hold bent position and take one full breath consisting of a slow, steady inhale and a slow, steady exhale. Return to neutral.

Benefits: Expands mobility in the back and strengthens the muscles of the lower back.

ALTERNATING ARM RAISES WITH WEIGHTS

Starting Position: Come to Mountain Pose holding the two-pound weights in your hands as they rest on your thighs.

Movement: Inhale as you lift your right arm above your head, only if this movement is pain free. If it isn't, then lift your arm as high as it will go comfortably. Try to keep your extended arm straight and your shoulder relaxed. Exhale as you lower your arm down. Switch sides.

Repetitions: Repeat six times on each side. Hold the pose on the last rep of each side and take one full breath. Release pose and return to neutral. You are holding the weights in both hands throughout the exercise.

Benefits: Lubricates the shoulder joint and strengthens the arms.

Let's pause and take three full breaths. Inhale slow and steady through your nose, and exhale slow and steady out your mouth.

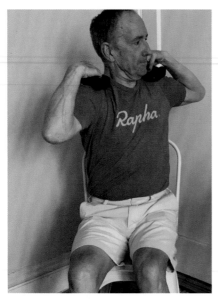

Torso Twist with Weights on Shoulders

TORSO TWIST WITH WEIGHTS ON SHOULDERS

Starting Position: Assume the Mountain Pose with weights in each hand and place your hands on your shoulders.

Movement: On an inhale, twist slowly to your right. Your head travels with your right arm. Exhale back to neutral. Don't lower your arms. Inhale and twist to your left. Your head travels with your left arm. Return to neutral and bring your arms down with hands resting on your legs.

Repetitions: Repeat each set eight times. Hold the pose on the last rep on each side and take two full breaths. Release the pose and return to neutral.

Benefits: Tones waistline and strengthens arms.

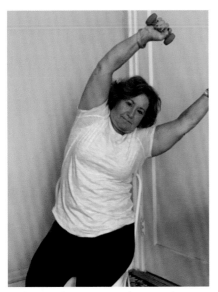

Side Body Lean with Weights

SIDE BODY LEAN WITH WEIGHTS

Starting Position: Sit up nice and tall in Mountain Pose. Take weights in each hand and rest them on your thighs.

Movement: With weights in both hands, inhale as you lift both arms up and stay. Exhale. On your next inhale, lean to your right. Exhale as you bring your arms back up to neutral. On a slow, steady inhale, with arms still up over your head, lean to your left. Exhale as you lift both arms up overhead.

Repetitions: Do eight sets. Arms stay up throughout. On the last rep on each side, hold the pose and take two full breaths. Release the pose and return to neutral.

Benefits: Tones waistline.

BICEP CURLS ALTERNATING ARMS WITH WEIGHTS

Starting Position: Come to sit in Mountain Pose with the weights in your hands.

Movement: Drop your arms by your sides. Keep your elbows glued to the sides of your body. On the inhale, slowly bend your right arm up and exhale as you lower it down to starting position. Inhale as you bring the left arm up and exhale to bring it back to start. Your elbows never leave the sides of your torso during the movement.

Repetitions: Repeat eight times on each side. Pause for a breath and repeat the exercise for eight reps on each side.

Benefits: Builds muscle in the biceps.

Bicep Curls Alternating Arms with Weights

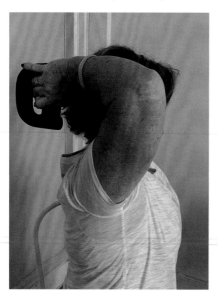

Overhead Tricep Curls with Weights

OVERHEAD TRICEP CURLS WITH WEIGHTS

Starting Position: Come to sit in Mountain Pose.

Movement: Hold one weight overhead with both hands, with a slight bend in your elbows. Inhale. On the exhale, lower your hands toward your upper back, keeping your forearms parallel with the floor and your elbows close to your head. Inhale to extend your hands back up to the overhead position. Exhale.

Repetitions: Do six sets of this exercise. Return to resting Mountain Pose. Take two full breaths and repeat the six sets.

Benefits: Strengthens triceps and upper back.

Let's pause again and take three full breaths. Inhale slow and steady through your nose, and exhale slow and steady out your mouth.

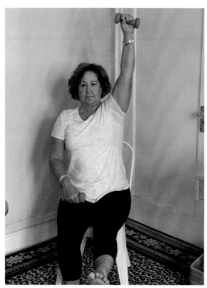

Single Arm and Leg Raises with Weights

SINGLE ARM AND LEG RAISES WITH WEIGHTS

Starting Position: Come to Mountain Pose with weights resting in your lap.

Movement: Inhale as you lift your right arm (weight is in your hand) and right leg together. Both your arm and leg should be as straight as you can make them. Exhale as you lower them.

Repetitions: Repeat six times on each side. Hold pose in the up position on the last rep of each side and take two full breaths. Release the pose and return to neutral.

Benefits: Strengthens arm and leg muscles. Expands coordination.

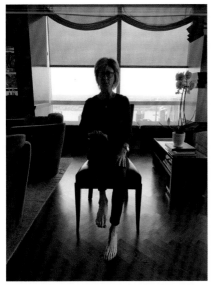

Single Knee Raises with Weights

SINGLE KNEE RAISES WITH WEIGHTS

Starting Position: Sit up tall in Mountain Pose with both weights resting on the top of your right knee.

Movement: Resting your right hand over the two weights to hold them in place, slowly lift your right knee straight up and then slowly lower your foot to the floor. Repeat ten times. On the final rep, hold your knee up and take two full breaths. Return your foot to the floor and switch sides. Place the two weights on top of your left knee.

Repetitions: Repeat ten times on each side. Make sure that you take two full breaths on the last rep of each side. Release pose.

Benefits: Strengthens quadriceps.

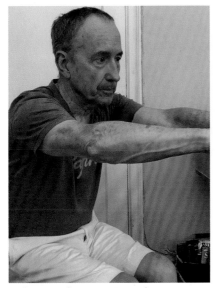

Advanced Sit to Stand

ADVANCED SIT TO STAND

Starting Position: Sit up tall in your chair.

Movement: Bend forward slightly, with your back straight, and look straight ahead. Extend your arms straight out in front. Now lift up out of the chair and stand tall and immediately sit back down. Keep your arms extended.

Repetitions: Repeat the movement eight times, quickly. Rest for a breath and repeat eight times, slowly.

Benefits: Builds strength overall, especially in your gluteus muscles, and improves balance. Also strengthens the core.

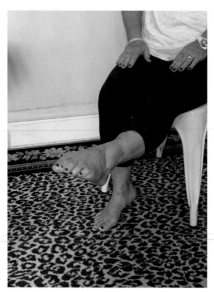

Single Leg Point and Flex

SINGLE LEG POINT AND FLEX

Starting Position: Sit tall in your chair with a straight spine.

Movement: On an inhale, extend your right leg straight out in front of you. Keeping your leg in this position, begin to point and flex your right foot. This can be done slowly or quickly. Either way, your foot and ankle get a terrific workout. Place your hands anywhere it is comfortable, whether that is down by your sides or in your lap. If possible, exaggerate both the point and the flex. When finished, return your foot to the floor and switch sides.

Repetitions: Repeat fifteen times on each side.

Benefits: Stretches shin and calf muscles while working the foot and ankle.

SINGLE LEG ANKLE CIRCLES

Starting Position: Sit tall in your chair in Mountain Pose.

Movement: Inhale as you lift your right leg up and begin to rotate your foot clockwise. Slowly articulate the circles. Make them as big and exaggerated as possible. After about ten rotations, switch direction. Keep your lifted leg as straight as possible. Switch legs.

Repetitions: Ten sets each side.

Benefits: Promotes mobility in and strengthens ankles.

Single Leg Ankle Circles

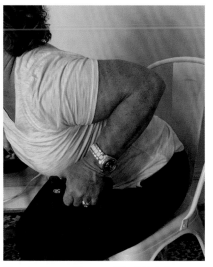

Bent Over Row with Weights

BENT OVER ROW WITH WEIGHTS

Starting Position: Come to Mountain Pose with weights in hands, resting on top of your legs.

Movement: Bend forward from hips with a straight back. Look straight ahead. On an inhale, pull your elbows back, keeping arms close to the sides of your body. On the exhale, slowly lower your arms all the way down. Keep your arms straight and stay in the bent forward position. On an inhale, slowly pull your arms all the way back up. At the top of the pose, your hands will be at the sides of your chest. Exhale to lower your arms down to the straight arms position. Remember to keep a straight back, forward bend position throughout the exercise while always looking straight ahead.

Repetitions: Do six sets. Pause for two full breaths, then repeat the six sets.

Benefits: Strengthens upper back, lower back, and biceps.

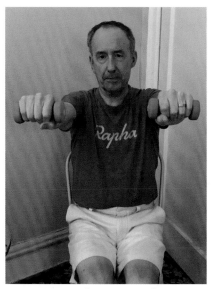

Arms Up and Down with Weights

ARMS UP/ARMS DOWN, ARMS OPEN/ARMS CLOSED WITH WEIGHTS

Starting Position: Come to sit tall in your chair. Belly button to spine. Weights in hands, resting in your lap.

Movement: On an inhale, extend your arms straight out in front. Exhale. On the inhale, lift arms up overhead and exhale them back to straight out in front. Inhale to open your straight arms out to the side, exhale to bring them back to straight out in front. Lower arms to Mountain Pose. This movement is one set. An easy way

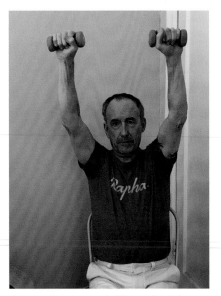

Arms Open and Closed with Weights

to remember the steps once you extend your arm out in front is to say: up, down, open, close.

Repetitions: Do six sets. Rest for two breaths and repeat.

Benefits: Builds stamina and upper body strength.

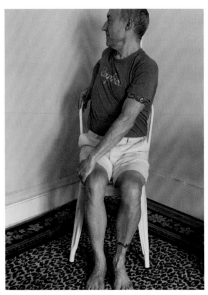

Chair Twist

CHAIR TWIST

Starting Position: Sit tall with feet hip distance apart.

Movement: Slowly twist your upper torso to your right and put your right hand on the top of the back of the chair. Place your left hand on the outside of your right knee. Make sure that both of your knees are pointing straight ahead. On an inhale, lift your spine and then exhale as you slowly twist to the right. Come back to neutral. This pose takes some practice. Do make sure that your lower body stays still!

Repetitions: Repeat five times on each side.

Benefits: Massages internal organs and tones the waistline.

BACK BEND

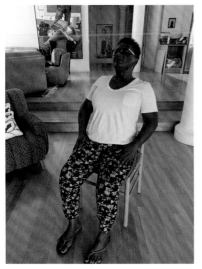

Back Bend

Starting Position: Come to Mountain Pose.

Movement: Rest your hands with your palms down on your legs. On a slow, steady inhale, lift your chest, arch your back slightly, open up your shoulders, and gaze up to the ceiling. On your exhale, slowly drop your head, round your back and shoulders, and gaze down at the floor. Now return to neutral. Let's do that again. Make the four movements—lift chest, arch back, open shoulders, and gaze up—happen simultaneously on a single inhale and likewise on the exhale. This may take a bit of practice but is worth the effort.

Repetitions: Do five sets of this pose.

Benefits: Warms up the thoracic and lumbar spine (upper and lower back). Promotes good posture.

Let's pause again and take three full breaths. Inhale slow and steady through your nose, and exhale slow and steady out your mouth.

SINGLE LEG LIFTS WITH WEIGHTS

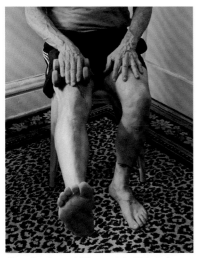

Single Leg Lifts with Weights

Starting Position: Sit tall in Mountain Pose and rest both weights on the top of your right thigh close to your knee.

Movement: Extend your right leg out and keep it as straight as possible. Rest your right hand over the two weights and slowly begin to lift your leg up from the chair in this position. Keep your back straight as you lift.

Repetitions: Lift your straight leg eight times on each side. On the eighth rep on each side, hold the uplifted leg for two full breaths. Release.

Benefits: Strengthens muscles in entire leg.

119

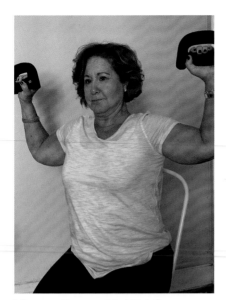

Victory Pose with Weights

VICTORY POSE WITH WEIGHTS

Starting Position: Sit tall in Mountain Pose with weights in your hands, resting in your lap.

Movement: Inhale as you lift your arms out to your sides with palms facing down. On an exhale bend your arms at the elbows. Your forearms will be perpendicular to your upper arms. The pose will look like a goal post. Check your alignment for straight spine, shoulders relaxed. Inhale to bring your arms toward one another, stopping when they are shoulder width apart, and keeping the position of parallel forearms. Exhale to return bent arms to the original position.

Repetitions: Repeat each rep six times. Return to resting Mountain Pose and take two full breaths. Repeat the exercise with six reps.

Benefits: Strengthens shoulders, arms, and upper back.

HEEL RAISES

Starting Position: Sit tall and point feet straight ahead.

Movement: Keeping toes firmly planted on the floor, begin to lift your heels. Keep lifting your heels, making sure that your toes remain on the floor. If it is comfortable to do so, exaggerate the heel lift each time.

Repetitions: Repeat fifteen times.

Benefits: Stretches your calf muscles.

Heel Raises

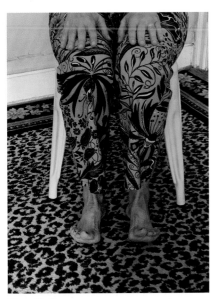
Toe Raises

TOE RAISES

Starting Position: Sit tall with feet pointed straight ahead.

Movement: Keeping heels firmly planted on the floor, begin to lift your toes. Keep lifting your toes while making certain that your heels remain firmly on the floor. Again, if it feels okay, exaggerate the lift each time.

Repetitions: Repeat fifteen times.

Benefits: Stretches the shins.

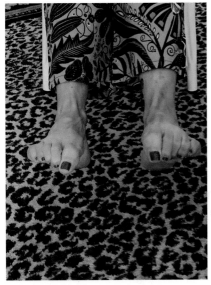
Toe Squeeze

TOE SQUEEZE/TOE SPREAD

Starting Position: Sit in Mountain Pose.

Movement: On an inhale, extend both legs out in front. Keep them there while you begin to scrunch your toes as tightly as you can, then release the squeeze and spread your toes out as widely as possible. Scrunch again, keeping everything tight, tight, tight! Then release and spread. Imagine that you can spread your toes so wide that no toe is touching another toe. This is really just a goal to work toward. Most likely, a toe or two will be touching.

Repetitions: Repeat this at least fifteen times. It feels good!

Benefits: Stretches toes, feet, and ankles.

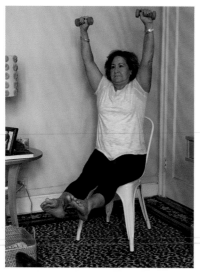

Everything Up with Weights

EVERYTHING UP WITH WEIGHTS!

Starting Position: This is your final Mountain Pose for this thirty-minute chair yoga workout. Make it a good one. Sit tall, knees hip distance apart, with toes pointing straight ahead. Keep your belly to spine. Hold weights in each hand and rest them on your legs.

Movement: On an inhale, lift your arms and legs up at the same time. Weights are in your hands. Try to keep all limbs and your back as straight as comfort will allow. Exhale, and slowly return arms and legs to starting position.

Repetitions: Repeat this pose eight times. On the last rep, hold the pose and take two full breaths. Release.

Benefits: Strengthens full body.

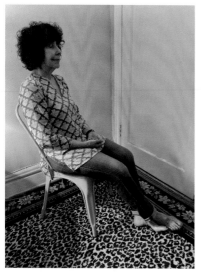

Deep Relaxation Pose

DEEP RELAXATION POSE

Starting Position: Lean back, resting your spine against the chair. Place your hands comfortably in your lap and close your eyes.

Movement: Breathe easily and relax your whole body. Allow any tension in your face, shoulders, legs, and feet to release.

Repetitions: Stay in this relaxed position for about five minutes, continuing to breathe naturally.

Benefits: Allows your body to absorb all of the benefits of your yoga practice.

Now that you have spent thirty minutes making your body stronger and more flexible, why not take an additional five to ten minutes to meditate.

CHAPTER THIRTEEN

BEGINNER PROGRAM FOR OSTEOARTHRITIS OF THE HANDS, KNEES, AND HIPS

According to the Arthritis Foundation, exercise is considered to be the most effective non-drug treatment for reducing pain and improving movement in osteoarthritis. A fear of pain and of causing further harm to the joints stops many individuals affected by osteoarthritis from exercising.

The main characteristics of osteoarthritis are pain, stiffness, and swelling caused by degeneration of the cartilage and bones within a joint. The knees, hips, and hands are most frequently affected. More than one in three adults sixty-two and older are affected.

Counterintuitively, aching joints are less painful when you are active. Exercise strengthens the muscles that support the joints, keeps the joints lubricated, and prevents the muscles and tendons from stiffening.

Three kinds of exercise are important for people with osteoarthritis: exercises involving range of motion (also called flexibility exercises), strengthening exercises, and aerobic exercises. We will focus on flexibility and strengthening poses. Please consult your physician or physical therapist before undertaking any aerobic exercise.

A recent study published in the Journal of American Geriatrics Society tested the effects of chair yoga on osteoarthritis and found it to be a safe and effective alternative pain management solution for aging adults with the condition. Study participants attended chair yoga sessions two times a week for eight weeks. Pain, gait speed, fatigue, and functional ability were all measured. After the eight weeks, participants showed significant improvement on all measures.

In an interview with *Practical Pain Management* magazine, Dr. Joseph Ruane, a highly rated sports medicine specialist, explained how yoga can help people with osteoarthritis manage their pain. "Motion is lotion for arthritis," says Dr. Ruane. "I often guide patients in my practice toward exercises like yoga because they are safe and helpful. Yoga not only improves strength and flexibility but it also helps them overcome a fear of falling."

Are you convinced yet? I hope so. Let's give this a go. For the beginner program, I'd like you to think of the entire twenty minutes as a full body warm-up.

I want to remind you of a few items on our getting started checklist:

- Drink a glass of water.
- Dress comfortably.
- Have your favorite music ready to go.
- Place your chair in an uncluttered space.
- Be barefoot or wear rubber-soled shoes on any floor surface. Wear socks only on carpet.
- Place this book on your music stand. It is really helpful to have book at eye level.

We will start with your neck and move down the body, ending with your feet.

NECK AND HEAD WARM-UPS

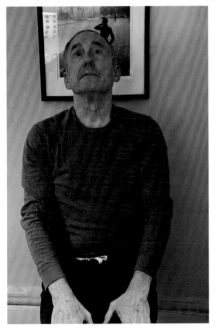

Upward and Downward Neck Stretch

UPWARD AND DOWNWARD NECK STRETCH

Starting Position: Come to Mountain Pose position. Sit up tall in your chair, shoulders back slightly, feet a few inches apart and pointed straight ahead. Rest your hands on top of your thighs.

Movement: On a slow and steady inhale, lift your head and gaze at the ceiling. As you slowly exhale, glide your head downward, chin to chest. Be as slow and gentle as possible with your movement.

Repetitions: Repeat this pose six times.

Benefits: Warms up and gently stretches the front and back of your neck.

NECK TURNS

Starting Position: Return to Mountain Pose.

Movement: On an inhale, very slowly turn your head to the right. As you exhale, very slowly return to center. On an inhale, turn your head slowly to the left. On a slow and steady exhale, return to center.

Repetitions: Repeat the set three times.

Benefits: Eases tension in the neck and helps to restore mobility in the upper back.

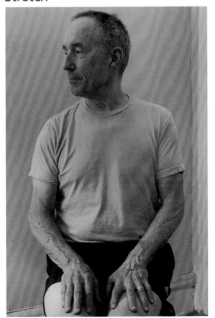

Neck Turns

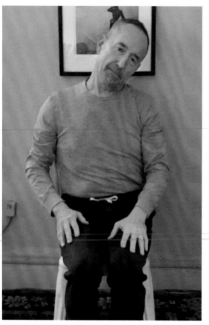

Side Neck Bend

SIDE NECK BEND

Starting Position: Come to Mountain Pose.

Movement: Inhale to sit tall. As you exhale, drop your right ear to your right shoulder. Make sure that your shoulders are relaxed. Inhale to bring your head back to neutral. Now inhale to sit tall and exhale as you bring your left ear to your left shoulder. Inhale to bring your head back to neutral. That is one set.

Repetitions: Repeat each set six times.

Benefits: Stretches the sides of the neck.

We are ready to move on to our shoulders. We hold so much tension in our shoulders and upper back, which is why it is so important to relax this area of our body. We can do that by gently warming up the surrounding muscles.

SHOULDER AND ARM WARM-UPS

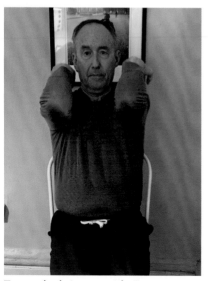

Extended Arms with Bent Elbows

EXTENDED ARMS WITH BENT ELBOWS

Starting Position: Come to sit in Mountain Pose.

Movement: Extend both arms straight out in front of you. Do this as comfortably as you can. Keep your shoulders down, as they tend to creep up during this pose. Make soft fists with your hands. Bend your forearms back so your soft fists touch your shoulders. Your upper arms remain parallel to the floor. Return your arms to starting position.

Repetitions: Repeat this movement ten times. Move slowly throughout.

Benefits: Lubricates and releases tension in shoulders.

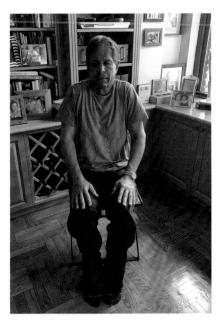

Shoulder Shrugs

SHOULDER SHRUGS

Starting Position: Resume Mountain Pose.

Movement: Inhale as you bring both shoulders up to your ears and exhale as you bring them back to neutral. Exaggerate the lift.

Repetitions: Repeat five times.

Benefits: Eases muscle tension in the neck and shoulders.

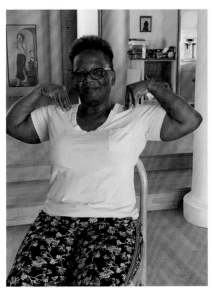

Hands on Shoulders Rolls

HANDS ON SHOULDERS ROLLS

Starting Position: Begin in Mountain Pose.

Movement: Place your hands on your shoulders and begin to make large circles with your shoulders, leading with your elbows. Breathe comfortably as you move. Switch the direction of your circles.

Repetitions: Repeat eight times in each direction.

Benefits: Warms up the upper back and releases tension in your neck.

FLIES WITH HANDS ON SHOULDERS

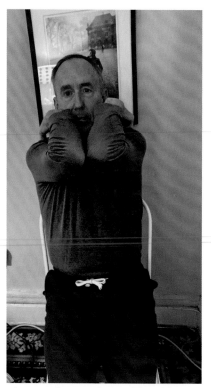

Flies with Hands on Shoulders

Starting Position: Begin this exercise in Mountain Pose.

Movement: Bring your hands to your shoulders and raise your elbows until your upper arms are parallel with the floor. On an inhale, bring your elbows to meet in front of your chest, or as close as you can bring your elbows together. On the exhale, open your elbows out to the sides of your body, keeping them at shoulder height. On each of the movements keep your pace slow, as well as your breaths.

Repetitions: Repeat each set six times. Return to Mountain Pose, take two slow and steady breaths, and repeat movement six times.

Benefits: Stretches upper back while releasing tension.

Let's now move on to our hands. As we age most of us will experience some form of arthritis in our hands, wrists, and fingers. The next three poses are very effective in maintaining function.

HAND WARM-UPS

WRIST AND HAND STRETCH

Starting Position: Sit up tall with a straight spine.

Movement: Extend both of your arms straight out in front of you, parallel to the floor. Make sure that your shoulders are down and relaxed. On the inhale, draw your hands back, bending at the wrist, so that all of your fingers point upwards. Exaggerate the

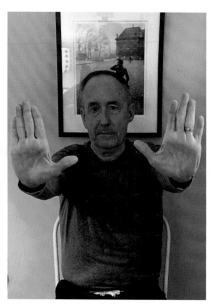

Wrist and Hand Stretch

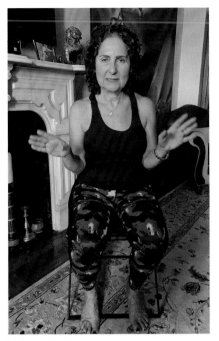

Wrist Circles

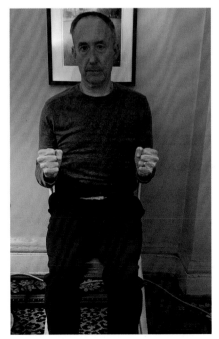

Finger Squeeze

upward extension. As you exhale, bend at the wrist so that your hands and fingers point downwards. Keep your arms extended throughout.

Repetitions: Repeat each set ten times.

Benefits: Deep stretch in wrists and hands.

WRIST CIRCLES

Starting Position: Sit up tall in Mountain Pose. Sit with belly to spine and the crown of your head lifted toward the ceiling.

Movement: Keep your elbows close to the sides of your body and extend your hands in front of you. With fingers extended, roll your hands at the wrists. Wiggle your fingers as you roll your wrists.

Repetitions: Roll your wrists ten times, then switch direction and roll again ten times.

Benefits: Warms up the wrists and fingers. Also relieves inflammation in the hand joints.

FINGER SQUEEZE

Starting Position: Sit up tall in Mountain Pose.

Movement: Bring your elbows into your waist and make soft fists with your hands. Squeeze your fists as tight as you can then open up your hands, extending fingers as straight as possible. Breathe naturally during this exercise.

Repetitions: Repeat this movement twenty times.

Benefits: Warms up the finger joints, giving them much needed lubrication.

We are ready to move on to our knees.

KNEE WARM-UPS

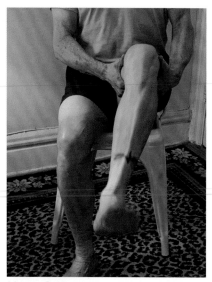

Knee Swings

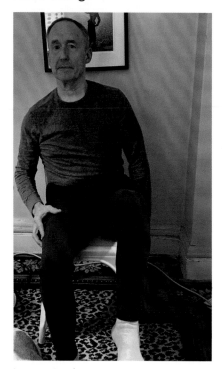

Knee Circles

KNEE SWINGS

Starting Position: Sit up tall in Mountain Pose, with belly in and shoulders back.

Movement: Clasp your hands under your right knee. Sit up tall with a straight spine. While holding under your knee, start to kick your leg out back and forth. Start out slowly and try the full range of motion. If you are unable to reach under your knee, then sit back in the chair and kick out your right leg, back and forth with as full range of motion as possible.

Repetitions: Do twenty times for each leg.

Benefits: Increases mobility and range of motion in the knees.

KNEE CIRCLES

Starting Position: Sit up tall in your chair with a straight spine.

Movement: Lift your right knee straight up, about six inches off the floor. Begin to make small, slow circles with your knee. Make sure that your left hip doesn't ride up while you are circling your right knee. After six rotations, reverse direction for six circles. Breathe naturally throughout movement. Return right foot to the floor and repeat the exercise for the left knee.

Repetitions: Repeat each set of exercises three times for each knee.

Benefits: Lubricates knee joint and releases tension in the knees.

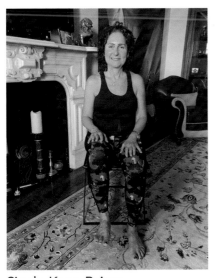

Single Knee Raises

SINGLE KNEE RAISES

Starting Position: Sit up tall in Mountain Pose.

Movement: Slowly lift your right knee straight up and slowly lower your foot to the floor. Lift your knee as high as you are able.

Repetitions: Repeat ten times on each side.

Benefits: Strengthens quadriceps.

Now let's move down the body to the feet.

FEET WARM-UPS

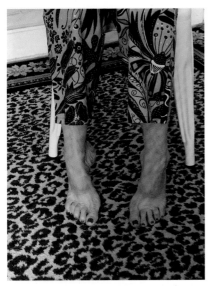

Heel Raises

HEEL RAISES

Starting Position: Sit tall and point feet straight ahead.

Movement: Keeping toes firmly planted on the floor, begin to lift your heels. Keep lifting your heels, making sure that your toes remain on the floor. If it is comfortable to do so, exaggerate the heel lift each time.

Repetitions: Repeat fifteen times.

Benefits: Stretches your calf muscles.

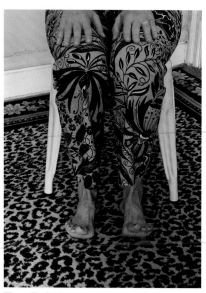

Toe Raises

TOE RAISES

Starting Position: Sit tall with feet pointed straight ahead.

Movement: Keeping heels firmly planted on the floor, begin to lift your toes. Keep lifting your toes while making certain that your heels remain firmly on the floor. Again, if it feels okay, exaggerate the lift each time.

Repetitions: Repeat fifteen times.

Benefits: Stretches the shins.

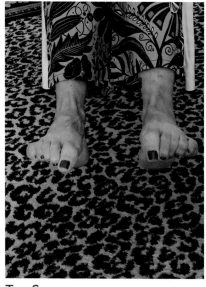

Toe Squeeze

TOE SQUEEZE/TOE SPREAD

Starting Position: Sit in Mountain Pose.

Movement: On an inhale, extend both legs out in front. Keep them there while you begin to scrunch your toes as tightly as you can, then release the squeeze and spread your toes out as widely as possible. If it is uncomfortable to keep your legs lifted, do this with your heels on the floor and your toes extended up. Scrunch again, keeping everything tight, tight, tight! Then release and spread. Imagine that you can spread your toes so wide that no toe is touching another toe. This is really just a goal to work toward. Most likely, a toe or two will be touching.

Repetitions: Repeat this at least fifteen times. It feels good!

Benefits: Stretches toes, feet, and ankles.

SINGLE LEG POINT AND FLEX

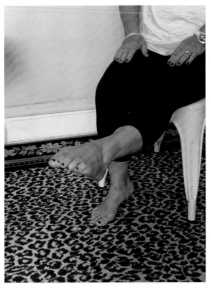

Single Leg Point and Flex

Starting Position: Sit tall in your chair with a straight spine.

Movement: On an inhale, extend your right leg straight out in front of you. Keeping your right leg in this position, begin to point and flex your right foot. As with the toe squeeze, if it is uncomfortable to keep your legs extended then do this pose with your heels on the floor and toes pointed up. Place your hands anywhere it is comfortable, whether that is down by your sides or in your lap. If possible, exaggerate both the point and the flex. When finished, return your foot to the floor and switch sides. Breathe naturally throughout.

Repetitions: Repeat fifteen times on each side.

Benefits: Stretches shin and calf muscles while also working the foot and ankle.

SINGLE LEG ANKLE CIRCLES

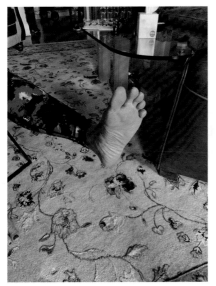

Single Leg Ankle Circles

Starting Position: Sit tall in your chair in Mountain Pose.

Movement: Inhale as you lift your right leg up and begin to rotate your foot clockwise. Slowly articulate the circles. Make them as big and exaggerated as possible. After about ten rotations, switch direction. Keep your lifted leg as straight as possible. Switch legs.

Repetitions: Ten sets each side.

Benefits: Promotes mobility in and strengthens ankles.

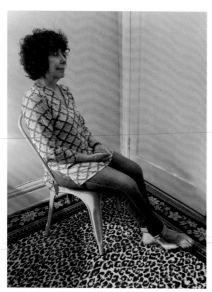

Deep Relaxation Pose

DEEP RELAXATION POSE

Starting Position: Lean back, resting your spine against the chair. Place your hands comfortably in your lap and close your eyes.

Movement: Breathe easily and relax your whole body. Allow any tension in your face, shoulders, legs, and feet to release.

Repetitions: Stay in this relaxed position for about five minutes, continuing to breathe naturally.

Benefits: Allows your body to absorb all of the benefits of your yoga practice.

You're finished! I hope that you feel relaxed and your muscles and joints feel fluid and ready to move. Please do try to do this routine three to five times a week. I believe if you do this for a few weeks you will be ready to move on to the next chapter of the osteoarthritis yoga routine. It is considered intermediate because we incorporate light weights to help maintain and build muscle strength. Are you ready to give it a shot?

CHAPTER FOURTEEN

INTERMEDIATE PROGRAM FOR OSTEOARTHRITIS OF THE HANDS, KNEES, AND HIPS

The only additional equipment needed for this workout compared to the Beginner Program for Osteoarthritis is a pair of lightweight dumbbells. We can start with two-pounds each and if and when you feel ready, we can move up to three- or four-pounds for each dumbbell.

Before we start with the weight bearing poses, let's start with the warm-up sequence that we did in the beginner's program.

NECK AND HEAD WARM-UPS

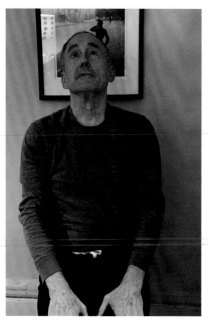

Upward and Downward Neck Stretch

UPWARD AND DOWNWARD NECK STRETCH

Starting Position: Come to Mountain Pose position. Sit up tall in your chair, shoulders back slightly, feet a few inches apart and pointed straight ahead. Rest your hands on top of your thighs.

Movement: On a slow and steady inhale, lift your head and gaze at the ceiling. As you slowly exhale, glide your head downward, chin to chest. Be as slow and gentle as possible with your movement.

Repetitions: Repeat this pose six times.

Benefits: Warms up and gently stretches the front and back of your neck.

NECK TURNS

Starting Position: Return to Mountain Pose.

Movement: On an inhale, very slowly turn your head to the right. As you exhale, very slowly return to center. On an inhale, turn your head slowly to the left. On a slow and steady exhale, return to center.

Repetitions: Repeat the set six times.

Benefits: Eases tension in the neck and helps to restore mobility in the upper back.

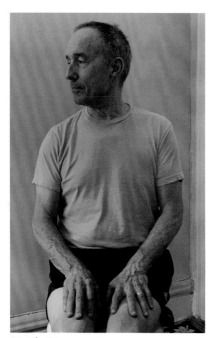

Neck Turns

SIDE NECK BEND

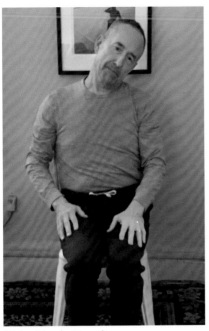

Side Neck Bend

Starting Position: Come to Mountain Pose.

Movement: Inhale to sit tall. As you exhale, drop your right ear to your right shoulder. Make sure that your shoulders are relaxed. Inhale to bring your head back to neutral. Now inhale to sit tall and exhale as you bring your left ear to your left shoulder. Inhale to bring your head back to neutral. That is one set.

Repetitions: Repeat each set six times.

Benefits: Stretches the sides of the neck.

We are ready to move on to our shoulders. We hold so much tension in our shoulders and upper back, which is why it is so important to relax this area of our body. We can do that by gently warming up the surrounding muscles.

SHOULDER AND ARM WARM-UPS

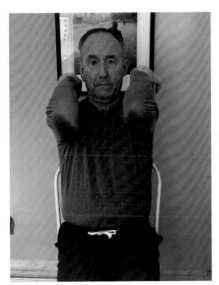

Extended Arms with Bent Elbows

EXTENDED ARMS WITH BENT ELBOWS

Starting Position: Come to sit in Mountain Pose.

Movement: Extend both arms straight out in front of you. Do this as comfortably as you can. Keep your shoulders down, as they tend to creep up during this pose. Make soft fists with your hands. Bend your forearms back so your soft fists touch your shoulders. Your upper arms remain parallel to the floor. Return your arms to starting position.

Repetitions: Repeat this movement ten times. Move slowly throughout.

Benefits: Lubricates and releases tension in shoulders.

137

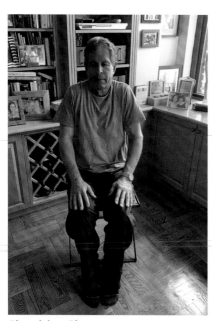

Shoulder Shrugs

SHOULDER SHRUGS

Starting Position: Resume Mountain Pose.

Movement: Inhale as you bring both shoulders up to your ears and exhale as you bring them back to neutral. Exaggerate the lift.

Repetitions: Repeat five times.

Benefits: Eases muscle tension in the neck and shoulders.

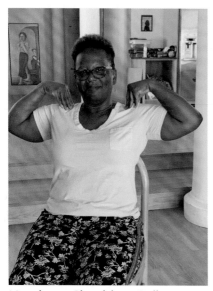

Hands on Shoulders Rolls

HANDS ON SHOULDERS ROLLS

Starting Position: Begin in Mountain Pose.

Movement: Place your hands on your shoulders and begin to make large circles with your shoulders, leading with your elbows. Breathe comfortably as you move. Switch the direction of your circles.

Repetitions: Repeat eight times in each direction.

Benefits: Warms up the upper back and releases tension in your neck.

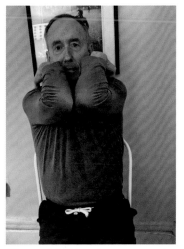

Flies with Hands on Shoulders

FLIES WITH HANDS ON SHOULDERS

Starting Position: Begin this exercise in Mountain Pose.

Movement: Bring your hands to your shoulders and raise your elbows until your upper arms are parallel with the floor. On an inhale, bring your elbows to meet in front of your chest, or as close as you can bring your elbows together. On the exhale, open your elbows out to the sides of your body, keeping them at shoulder height. On each of the movements, keep your pace slow, as well as your breaths.

Repetitions: Repeat each set six times. Return to Mountain Pose, take two slow and steady breaths, and repeat movement six times.

Benefits: Stretches upper back while releasing tension.

Let's now move on to our hands. As we age, most of us will experience some form of arthritis in our hands, wrists, and fingers. The next three poses are very effective in maintaining function.

HAND WARM-UPS

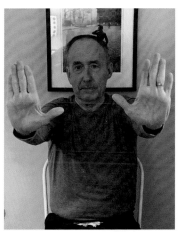

Wrist and Hand Stretch

WRIST AND HAND STRETCH

Starting Position: Sit up tall with a straight spine.

Movement: Extend both of your arms straight out in front of you, parallel to the floor. Make sure that your shoulders are down and relaxed. On the inhale, draw your hands back, bending at the wrist, so that all of your fingers point upwards. Exaggerate the upward extension. As you exhale, bend at the wrist so that your hands and fingers point downwards. Keep your arms extended throughout.

Repetitions: Repeat each set ten times.

Benefits: Deep stretch in wrists and hands.

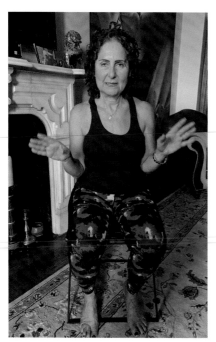

Wrist Circles

WRIST CIRCLES

Starting Position: Sit up tall in Mountain Pose. Sit with belly to spine and the crown of your head lifted toward the ceiling.

Movement: Keep your elbows close to the sides of your body and extend your hands in front of you. With fingers extended, roll your hands at the wrists. Wiggle your fingers as you roll your wrists.

Repetitions: Roll your wrists ten times, then switch direction and roll again ten times.

Benefits: Warms up the wrists and fingers. Also relieves inflammation in the hand joints.

FINGER SQUEEZE

Starting Position: Sit up tall in Mountain Pose.

Movement: Bring your elbows into your waist and make soft fists with your hands. Squeeze your fists as tight as you can then open up your hands, extending fingers as straight as possible. Breathe naturally during this exercise.

Repetitions: Repeat this movement twenty times.

Benefits: Warms up the finger joints, giving them much needed lubrication.

We are ready to move on to our knees.

Finger Squeeze

KNEE WARM-UPS

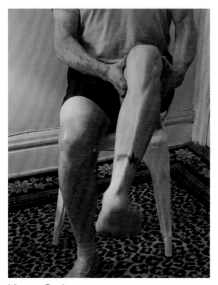

Knee Swings

KNEE SWINGS

Starting Position: Sit up tall in Mountain Pose, with belly in and shoulders back.

Movement: Clasp your hands under your right knee. Sit up tall with a straight spine. While holding under your knee, start to kick your leg out back and forth. Start out slowly and try the full range of motion. If you are unable to reach under your knee, then sit back in the chair and kick out your right leg, back and forth with as full range of motion as possible.

Repetitions: Do twenty times for each leg.

Benefits: Increases mobility and range of motion in the knees.

KNEE CIRCLES

Starting Position: Sit up tall in your chair with a straight spine.

Movement: Lift your right knee straight up, about six inches off the floor. Begin to make small, slow circles with your knee. Make sure that your left hip doesn't ride up while you are circling your right knee. After six rotations, reverse direction for six circles. Breathe naturally throughout movement. Return right foot to the floor and repeat the exercise for the left knee.

Repetitions: Repeat each set of exercises three times for each knee.

Benefits: Lubricates knee joint and releases tension in the knees.

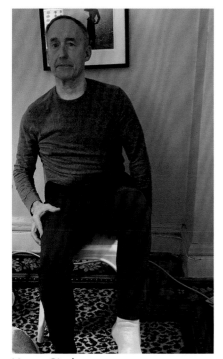

Knee Circles

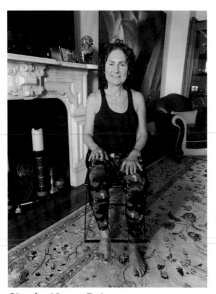

Single Knee Raises

SINGLE KNEE RAISES

Starting Position: Sit up tall in Mountain Pose.

Movement: Slowly lift your right knee straight up and slowly lower your foot to the floor. Lift your knee as high as you are able.

Repetitions: Repeat ten times on each side.

Benefits: Strengthens quadriceps.

Now let's move down the body to the feet.

FEET WARM-UPS

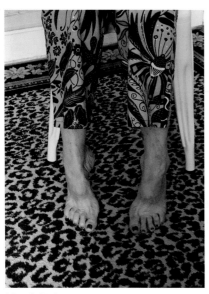

Heel Raises

HEEL RAISES

Starting Position: Sit tall and point feet straight ahead.

Movement: Keeping toes firmly planted on the floor, begin to lift your heels. Keep lifting your heels, making sure that your toes remain on the floor. If it is comfortable to do so, exaggerate the heel lift each time.

Repetitions: Repeat fifteen times.

Benefits: Stretches your calf muscles.

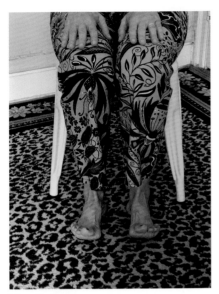

Toe Raises

TOE RAISES

Starting Position: Sit tall with feet pointed straight ahead.

Movement: Keeping heels firmly planted on the floor, begin to lift your toes. Keep lifting your toes while making certain that your heels remain firmly on the floor. Again, if it feels okay, exaggerate the lift each time.

Repetitions: Repeat fifteen times.

Benefits: Stretches the shins.

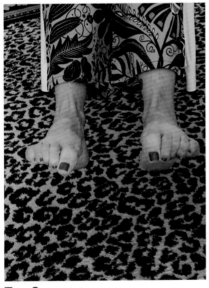

Toe Squeeze

TOE SQUEEZE/TOE SPREAD

Starting Position: Sit in Mountain Pose.

Movement: On an inhale, extend both legs out in front. Keep them there while you begin to scrunch your toes as tightly as you can, then release the squeeze and spread your toes out as widely as possible. If it is uncomfortable to keep your legs lifted, do this with your heels on the floor and your toes extended up. Scrunch again, keeping everything tight, tight, tight! Then release and spread. Imagine that you can spread your toes so wide that no toe is touching another toe. This is really just a goal to work toward. Most likely, a toe or two will be touching.

Repetitions: Repeat this at least fifteen times. It feels good!

Benefits: Stretches toes, feet, and ankles.

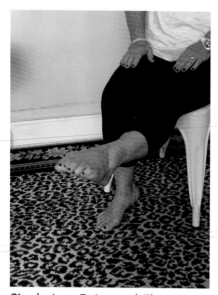

Single Leg Point and Flex

SINGLE LEG POINT AND FLEX

Starting Position: Sit tall in your chair with a straight spine.

Movement: On an inhale, extend your right leg straight out in front of you. Keeping your right leg in this position, begin to point and flex your right foot. As with the toe squeeze, if it is uncomfortable to keep your legs extended then do this pose with your heels on the floor and toes pointed up. Place your hands anywhere it is comfortable, whether that is down by your sides or in your lap. If possible, exaggerate both the point and the flex. When finished, return your foot to the floor and switch sides. Breathe naturally throughout.

Repetitions: Repeat fifteen times on each side.

Benefits: Stretches shin and calf muscles while also working the foot and ankle.

SINGLE LEG ANKLE CIRCLES

Starting Position: Sit tall in your chair in Mountain Pose.

Movement: Inhale as you lift your right leg up and begin to rotate your foot clockwise. Slowly articulate the circles. Make them as big and exaggerated as possible. After about ten rotations, switch direction. Keep your lifted leg as straight as possible. Switch legs.

Repetitions: Ten sets each side.

Benefits: Promotes mobility in and strengthens ankles.

Single Leg Ankle Circles

Time to work with your two-pound dumbbells. Start out gently. Stop doing these poses if they cause any pain or discomfort. The movements should be moderately challenging. Only you can determine when it is right to stop or pull back. Modifications can be made by reducing the number of recommended repetitions.

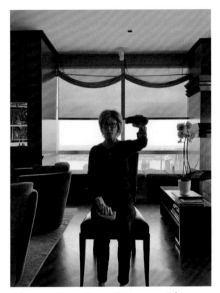

Alternating Arm Raises with Weights

ALTERNATING ARM RAISES WITH WEIGHTS

Starting Position: Come to Mountain Pose holding the two-pound weights in your hands as they rest on your thighs.

Movement: Inhale as you lift your right arm above your head, only if this movement is pain free. If it isn't, then lift your arm as high as it will go comfortably. Try to keep your extended arm straight and your shoulder relaxed. Exhale as you lower your arm down. Switch sides.

Repetitions: Repeat six times on each side. Hold the pose on the last rep of each side and take two full breaths. Release pose and return to neutral. You are holding the weights in both hands throughout the exercise.

Benefits: Lubricates the shoulder joint and strengthens the arms.

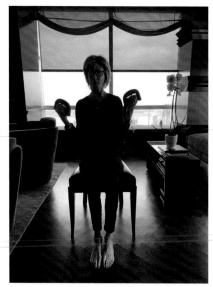

Bicep Curls Alternating Arms
with Weights

BICEP CURLS ALTERNATING ARMS WITH WEIGHTS

Starting Position: Come to sit in Mountain Pose with the weights in your hands.

Movement: Drop your arms by your sides. Keep your elbows glued to the sides of your body. On the inhale, slowly bend your right arm up and exhale as you lower it down to starting position. Inhale as you bring the left arm up and exhale to bring it back to start. Your elbows never leave the sides of your torso during the movement.

Repetitions: Repeat eight times on each side. Pause for a breath and repeat the exercise for eight reps on each side.

Benefits: Builds muscle in the biceps.

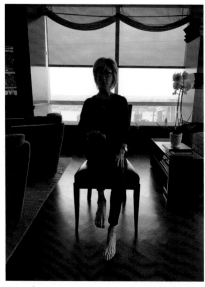

Single Knee Raises with Weights

SINGLE KNEE RAISES WITH WEIGHTS

Starting Position: Sit up tall in Mountain Pose with both weights resting on the top of your right knee.

Movement: Resting your right hand over the two weights to hold them in place, slowly lift your right knee straight up and then slowly lower your foot to the floor. Repeat ten times. Switch sides. Place the two weights on top of your left knee.

Repetitions: Repeat ten times on each side.

Benefits: Strengthens quadriceps.

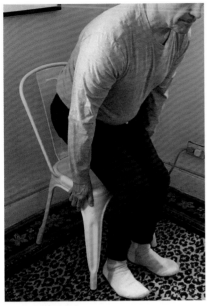

Sit to Stand

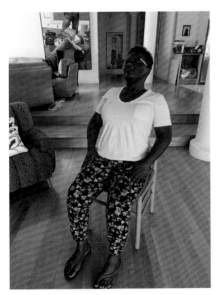

Back Bend

SIT TO STAND

Starting Position: Sit up tall in your chair.

Movement: Place your hands on the sides of the seat of the chair. Bend forward slightly with your back straight and look straight ahead. Now lift up out of the chair about six inches and then sit back down.

Repetitions: Repeat the movement eight times. If this is easy to do, then try extending your arms straight out in front of you as you elevate out of the chair.

Benefits: Builds strength in your gluteus muscles, which are the muscles that control sitting down and standing up. Improves overall balance.

BACK BEND

Starting Position: Come to Mountain Pose.

Movement: Rest your hands with your palms down on your legs. On a slow, steady inhale, lift your chest, arch your back slightly, open up your shoulders, and gaze up to the ceiling. On your exhale, slowly drop your head, round your back and shoulders, and gaze down at the floor. Now return to neutral. Let's do that again. Make the four movements—lift chest, arch back, open shoulders, and gaze up—happen simultaneously on a single inhale and likewise on the exhale. This may take a bit of practice but is worth the effort.

Repetitions: Do five sets of this pose.

Benefits: Warms up the thoracic and lumbar spine (upper and lower back). Promotes good posture.

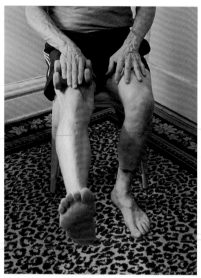

Single Leg Lifts with Weights

SINGLE LEG LIFTS WITH WEIGHTS

Starting Position: Sit tall in Mountain Pose and rest both weights on the top of your right thigh close to your knee.

Movement: Extend your right leg out and keep it as straight as possible. Rest your right hand over the two weights and slowly begin to lift your leg up from the chair in this position. Keep your back straight as you lift.

Repetitions: Lift your straight leg eight times on each side. On the eighth rep on each side, hold the uplifted leg for two full breaths. Release.

Benefits: Strengthens muscles in entire leg.

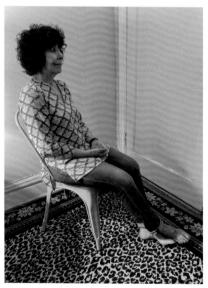

Deep Relaxation Pose

DEEP RELAXATION POSE

Starting Position: Lean back, resting your spine against the chair. Place your hands comfortably in your lap and close your eyes.

Movement: Breathe easily and relax your whole body. Allow any tension in your face, shoulders, legs, and feet to release.

Repetitions: Stay in this relaxed position for about five minutes, continuing to breathe naturally.

Benefits: Allows your body to absorb all of the benefits of your yoga practice.

Don't let aching joints hold you back anymore. Please pick the arthritis routine that works best for you. If you only ever do the beginner program, make sure that you do it often. Very often. The more you do it the better you will move and feel.

You have come to the end of this book. My hope is that you have tried the programs and found them to be helpful and enjoyable while also challenging. I encourage you to establish an exercise habit and stick with it.

You are on a wonderful journey that will afford you the opportunity for a happier, healthier, and more purposeful life. I am honored that you allowed me to be your guide. You did all of the work. It wasn't easy. Be proud. Share your learning with others.

ACKNOWLEDGMENTS

I want to express my deep gratitude to all the teachers I have had the joy of learning from during my yoga journey. My very first teacher was Beryl Bender Birch, who taught Yoga for Runners at the NY Road Runners Club. I was an avid runner at the time and wanted to relieve the accumulating tightness in my leg muscles. After three weeks of class, I was so enamored that I sought out a yoga studio to explore further. It was the beginning of a decades-long journey.

I want to thank the most loving and joyous teacher I have ever known, Jillian Pransky. I will forever be grateful to Jason Brown who helped me learn to do a headstand. I was deathly afraid to go upside down and he taught me to conquer that fear.

The next teacher on my yoga path was Lakshmi Voelker, who instructed me on how to teach chair yoga.

Thank you to Elizabeth Hartowicz, Director of the Care Program for older adults living with dementia at the Lenox Hill Neighborhood House, who gave me my very first gig as a chair yoga teacher. My forever thank you to my many clients. Each one of you has taught me to become a better teacher.

I would like to thank my dear friends who modeled for me for this book. They are: Hilarie Gopaul, David Lehmkuhl, Branche Lubart, Jane Newman, Lisa Reeves, Sandra Stark, Victor Santiago, and myself!

Finally, I want to acknowledge the five people who I get up in the morning for: David, Mia, Conor, Winona, and Luke. Thank you.